What people are saying about the RAVE Diet

"Just a quick line to give you some wonderful news. I no longer have prostate cancer – I am free of cancer at this time. I had a biopsy done on 10/3 and there is no evidence of cancer! The RAVE Diet book, the Eating DVD and the Healing Cancer DVD were instrumental in my recovery and healing." – Vincent Randazzo

"In just a few months, I have lost 32 pounds, my medications have been cut in half and my blood sugars, blood pressure and cholesterol have all dropped dramatically." – Sirmirrion English

"My husband is 59 years old and had a massive heart attack 3 years ago, quad bypass, 3 stents, defibrillator, diabetic (adult onset), horrid shingles, high blood pressure and before RAVE 205 pounds. Today, just 2 short months later, he is 180 pounds, off Metformin completely for his diabetes, off cholesterol medication and feeling better than when he was 35! One truly amazing thing is that he has not had one shingles outbreak since starting RAVE. For that alone he will be forever grateful for your research and putting it all in human terms!" – Susan Hoffmann

"My cholesterol dropped from 221 to 184. My blood pressure is 130 over 80, down from 150 over 98. My B-12, iron, sugar, calcium etc. were all perfect, and as an added bonus, I have lost 26 pounds over the course of the past 10 months. These are the best results I have ever had." – AnnMarie Iasimone

"I have lost 47 pounds over the past 12 months by changing my entire way of eating and following the RAVE Diet. This has helped me to not only lose the weight, but has also helped me to significantly lower my cholesterol, control my blood pressure, and better my self-esteem." – Albert J. Tarrano

"When I was 11 years old, I was diagnosed with cholesterol of 550. I have been to many different doctors and tried every kind of cholesterol lowering medication, but nothing worked. After following the RAVE diet, my cholesterol dropped to 400 points in just a few months. That is the lowest it has ever been – and without any medication. I was amazed! I've also lost 15 pounds and have never felt better." – Emily Burke

"My father has had numerous bypass surgeries (along with numerous other health related surgeries) and unfortunately must have the lower half of his leg amputated due to the artificial arteries becoming clogged (again) and no circulation occurring. After many years of him being on cholesterol lowering medication with no results, his cholesterol dropped 90 points in 3 weeks after starting the diet! In addition, he had a kidney transplant 1½ years ago and his creatin levels have always been high. Since starting the diet they too have dropped. His doctors were shocked and told him to just keep doing what he's doing!" – Christine Chiudina

The RAVE Diet

&

Lifestyle

by
Mike Anderson

Published by
www.RaveDiet.com

International Standard Book Number (ISBN)
978-0-9726590-6-2

First Edition: August 2004
Second Edition: September 2007
Third Edition: March 2009

Printed in the United States of America

For Harold, Virginia, Harvey and Reva, who suffered greatly from diet-related diseases, simply because they did not know any better.

Acknowledgments

Many people contributed to the making of this book, as well as the related film entitled *Eating*. I would like to thank the following individuals who volunteered their time and talented efforts to make both possible.

Reuben Allen
Zel Allen
Jesica Baker
Rosemary Byrne
Suzanne Cozens
John Hoffman
Matthew Israel
Valorie Kleiman
Jennifer Lee
Mark Lanier
Pedro Morales
Karen Porreca
Robyn Roth
Karen Van Sant
Terry Wayne
Judy Weber

Disclaimer

If you have any medical condition, you should change your diet only under the care of a physician. Neither the author nor any advisors for this book make any representation or warranty of any kind whatsoever regarding the appropriateness of this program for any individual. The information presented herein is not medical advice and is not given as medical advice. If you need a physician to work with you, please visit our web site at www.RaveDiet.com.

Forward

I became interested in diet many years ago, quite by accident. I had always thought I was eating a healthy diet, as did my family. Then some tragic events began to unfold. First, my father died of cancer. Next, my stepfather died of heart disease. Then my mother broke one hip and we discovered she had severe osteoporosis. Shortly thereafter, she broke her other hip. A friend of mine, who ate a "healthy" diet, discovered she had breast cancer. Just one year later, she suffered a heart attack.

As I moved into my late forties and passed the age of 50, it seemed like all my friends, family and relatives were suffering from one chronic disease or another. At that time, I more or less shrugged my shoulders and accepted this as a normal part of aging. Unfortunately, as I was to learn, it *is* a normal part of aging – but doesn't have to be.

At about the time I turned 50, I happened to pick up a book that declared, in no uncertain terms, that the major diseases in this country could be prevented and often reversed through diet and lifestyle changes. The corollary of that statement was that our major diseases were *caused* by diet and lifestyle.

I thought this was a pretty radical statement, but I was curious enough to read further and check out references that were provided within the book. One book led to another and another. In fact, I spent over two years, full-time, researching this subject and I've continued that research ever since.

Before my plunge into diet-related literature, I had always considered myself fairly well read yet I kept asking myself, "Why isn't this information more widely known?" Not only does the information linking diet and disease come from people with the highest credentials, but they have irrefutable evidence to back up their claims. "Why don't mainstream health authorities tell us about this? Why am I not reading about this in the newspapers?" Unfortunately, after years of research, I have the answer to that question, and it's not a pretty picture.

This information is so powerful that I felt compelled to share it with others, so they can make their own decisions based on *all* the facts. The first thing I did was to produce a film, entitled *Eating*. It turned out to be very powerful and has received much praise and attention. In fact, it is a life-changer for many people who watch it. There were many people, however, who needed more information and I received numerous requests to write a book that would provide more details about the subjects covered in *Eating*. The result was this book, *The RAVE Diet & Lifestyle*.

In the course of my research, I discovered there was a set of basic rules doctors used when arresting and reversing diseases with diet. These rules form the acronym RAVE. Doctors who reverse diseases with diet have their individual preferences and will emphasize certain foods over others, but all their diets fall within the RAVE concept.

Heart disease is the most documented and easily reversed disease in the books. But it's not just heart disease. Our common cancers – including breast, prostate, colon and other cancers, have not only been reversed, but can be totally prevented by following the RAVE Diet. Adult onset diabetes is a snap. One doctor gets 90 percent of his patients off insulin within a month by prescribing simple changes in diet. There are literally hundreds of other diseases, ranging from arthritis and autoimmune diseases to rheumatoid arthritis to shingles and varicose veins that can be arrested and reversed by following the RAVE Diet.

One of those diseases includes obesity, and its precursor, being overweight. I emphasize weight loss in this book because being overweight has, unfortunately, become "normal" in America. In fact, we've literally lost sight of what normal weight should be. It's become so bad that most people would consider someone at their ideal weight to be too skinny and sickly looking. Being overweight is a platform from which many diseases spring, so focusing on weight loss can bring a multitude of health benefits in its wake.

I know what some of you may be thinking: Reversing serious diseases with something as simple as diet may sound ludicrous. If you are thinking this, you're wearing the same shoes I found myself in years ago. I could not believe it, either, which is exactly why I felt compelled to help get this information out.

Some of you will consider my message radical, particularly if your dietary habits are within the mainstream. The irony is that I now consider "healthy" mainstream diets to be radical. After all, heart disease and our common cancers are the biggest killers in America today and they are the direct result of eating what most would consider a "healthy" mainstream diet. From the perspective of human history, the RAVE Diet is not a radical message at all. To advise that you follow a diet that reverses heart disease and prevents our common cancers is hardly radical. It's the most natural thing in the world. I hope that you won't consider my message radical, either, after you finish reading this book.

The reason I decided to put this information together is to present an easy-to-digest summary that will motivate people to change their diets in order to realize the dramatic health benefits that can result from such a simple, although ultimately profound, change in their lives. All families in America are being torn apart by diseases caused by the foods they eat. These diseases can not only be prevented, but also reversed, with simple changes in diet. Hopefully, you will try the RAVE Diet and reap the same health benefits many others have. It will turn your life into a happier existence, for not only yourself, but also your family, your friends and the world we all live in.

Mike Anderson

Introduction – The Tortoise and the Hare

"If everyone is thinking alike, then no one is thinking." – Benjamin Franklin

"Food is cheaper now by a long way, more abundantly available, more highly refined and more pressingly sold to us by very clever advertising companies and techniques. The remarkable thing is how anybody stays thin." – Dr. Andrew Prentice, London school of Hygiene and Tropical Medicine

Only in America do people order double cheeseburgers, large fries and a diet coke.

We live in a strange world when it comes to weight loss. Imagine, if you will, someone who's overweight giving advice on how to lose weight. Sounds ridiculous, right? Yet, what we have today are a bunch of fat doctors telling people how to lose weight. In fact, the most successful Diet Doctors seem to be the most overweight.

In the year 2000, long before the controversy about his weight after his death, Dr. Atkins exceeded federal guidelines for being overweight. One doctor, who saw him many times over the decades, estimated he was 40 to 60 pounds overweight.[1]

Barry Sears, Ph.D., author of the hugely popular Zone diet, was also overweight in the year 2000. Sears even states he's overweight in his own book![2] Yet despite this admission, millions of copies have been sold. Am I missing something? How can people who want to lose weight follow the advice of someone who proclaims, in his own book, that he's overweight?

Perhaps the answer lies in some of the statements that Sears makes, such as "You can burn more fat watching TV than by exercising"[3] and "About one-third of Americans are … suffering from protein malnutrition."[4] The last statement is like saying Americans are suffering from *fat* malnutrition. As a matter of fact, the average American eats enough protein to fuel a champion weight lifter. (See *Notes – Protein.*) But burning fat while watching TV and getting too little protein are the things Americans love to hear because it justifies eating the very diet that has made us the fattest nation on the planet.

---

[1] Attwood, Charles, M.D., "Enter the 'Zone': A Giant Leap Backwards" (1998). Many people, from the Mayor of New York City to other doctors who have known him for decades have all said that Atkins was overweight. Re Mayor Michael Bloomberg, Daily News, January 21, 2004. Dr. John McDougall estimates Atkins was 40 to 60 pounds overweight. Deborah Norville, MSNBC, 2/11/04.
[2] Barry Sears, Enter the Zone, p. 47.
[3] Barry Sears, Enter the Zone, pp. 3. 96, back cover.
[4] Barry Sears, Enter the Zone, pp. 67, 69.

We also have Dr. Phil, who at 6 foot 4 inches and 240 pounds is at the upper-end of the overweight category and teetering toward obesity, according to Harvard's Body Mass Index (BMI). And yet, he claims he's at an appropriate weight for his age and height.[5] By whose standard? And stating his weight as "age appropriate" implies that humans are supposed to gain weight with age, an obvious invention by Dr. Phil and his publicity machine. Of course, Dr. Phil also states that just about everyone can benefit from the supplements he's selling, particularly Dr. Phil.

Then again, other Diet Doctors are just plain terrified of their own diet. Look at Dr. Agatson, for example, author of the best-selling South Beach Diet. Here's a cardiologist who admits to taking an aspirin, fish oil capsules and a statin drug *every day* to prevent a heart attack.[6]

Imagine, if you will, a cardiologist who cannot even design a diet that will free him of drugs that treat a disease he's supposed to be an expert at preventing; a cardiologist who's incapable of designing a diet to lose weight *and* prevent heart disease. A cardiologist who says that eating a candy bar is healthier than eating a potato.[7] And while he tells his readers "Don't even think about limiting the amount of food you eat," his menu plans are, in fact, severely restricted in phase one. But, of course, if you start to gain weight in the later phases, you have to go back to his more restricted diet. In other words, he has a built-in yo-yo cycle within his own diet. And, there are no secrets. It's a simple calorie restriction diet, as are the Zone and Atkins diets. As Dr. Marion Nestle has stated, "What it comes down to is that this is a standard 1,200- to 1,400-calorie-a-day diet, so of course people are going to lose weight."[8]

Parenthetically, if you follow the South Beach Diet like its author, it's going to cost some $3,000 just in heart medicines, not to mention the aspirin and fish oil tablets. There are many doctors who design heart-healthy diets, they keep their total cholesterol well below 150 and they *do not* take aspirin, fish oil or any heart medicines, all of which can have serious side effects. Their healthy hearts are due solely to diet, not drugs. You can achieve far better results with diet than you can with drugs when it comes to heart disease, because no drug has ever *cured* heart disease whereas the RAVE Diet has.

Diet schemes have become so bad that we now have diets that are like nutritional astrology, such as the "dial a blood type" diet.[9] Since the majority of Americans are either type O or type B, the "blood type" diet has served as a way

---

[5] New York Times, 10/27/03.

[6] Doctor Wants 'South Beach' to Mean Hearts, Not Bikinis, New York Times, 4/14/04.

[7] This is based on using the dubious glycemic index. For more on this index, see *Notes – Problems With the Glycemic Index*.

[8] New York Times, 10/7/03.

[9] Eat Right 4 Your Type by Peter J. D'Adamo.

to justify gluttonous ways of eating and is similar to the Atkins' diet, for the O and B blood types.[10]

There are a number of things these popular diets have in common. Among them, they promise *immediate* weight loss. We're talking over a pound a day. Now, if that doesn't get the attention of someone desperate to lose weight, nothing will. And these books always have some unique, clever scheme, which is apparently unknown to the rest of the scientific world.

Unfortunately, the real world doesn't work that way. Despite claims that you can eat all you want, if you calculate the menu plans of these popular diet books, they're *all calorie restriction diets*!

After you get past the smoke and mirrors, it boils down to calories in, calories out. After an exhaustive analysis of some 107 diets, the American Medical Association found that all these popular diets had nothing to do with restricting carbohydrates and had everything to do with restricting calories.[11] Recently, a study confirmed what everyone should have known in the first place: The thinnest people in the world eat the highest amount of *complex* carbohydrates and the fattest people eat the highest amount of animal protein.[12]

Of course, these popular diets *do* work in the short-term. But then again, *any* calorie-restriction diet will work in the short term. You could eat nothing but lard and if you had fewer calories coming in than going out, you'd lose weight. The problem boils down to sticking with these bizarre diets in the long haul.

It seems when the going gets tough, doctors write diet books in order to make money. Every few years, the public is subjected to yet another "miracle diet" with some "secret" that will cause effortless weight loss. You purchase the book, follow the restricted dietary regimen and – almost miraculously – you're losing weight. Voila!

You're so proud of yourself, you tell your friends. And they're so impressed with your weight loss, they go out and buy a copy of the book, the supplements and whatever other gimmicks they're offering, all in an effort to save their waists and hiplines from seemingly perpetual expansion. And soon they begin telling all

---

[10] One example of why the blood type diet makes little sense: It posits that type B's should thrive on dairy products. This sounds great to Americans because the vast majority of white Americans (and Europeans) tolerate lactose (a sugar found in dairy products). On the other hand, the highest percentage of type B's in the world is found in Asia. But since 90 percent of Asians are lactose *intolerant* I can guarantee you they will not thrive on dairy products – just the opposite! Other gaping holes exist in the blood type theory. For an in-depth critique, see Michael Klapper, M.D., The Blood Type Diet: Fact or Fiction, at www.earthsave.org/news/bloodtyp.htm.

[11] Bravata DM, Sanders L, Huang J, et al., Efficacy and safety of low-carbohydrate diets: a systematic review. JAMA. 2003;289:1837-1850.

[12] Studies Link High-Fiber Carbs, Low Weight, WebMD Medical News, 3/5/04; American Heart Association Annual Conference on Cardiovascular Disease Epidemiology and Prevention, San Francisco, 2004.

their friends about the miracle diet that (finally!) took off those stubborn pounds. And so the circle of dieters grows as fast as the wallets of the Diet Doctors.

Now fast-forward just three years.

No one's talking any more.

In fact, 95 percent of the people who thought they had been saved from everlasting weight gain are off these strange diets.[13] Not only did the weight return, but they're heavier now than when they started the diet and they've increased their percentage of body fat to boot.

Some miracle.

They would have been better off had they never started the diet in the first place. In fact, research shows that dieters gain more weight in the long run than those who don't follow any weight-loss diet at all.

Now fast-forward just five years.

Virtually everyone who started the miracle diet is off the diet. In fact, it's a miracle they could put up with these eating regimens for so long.

The yo-yo diet cycle is nothing new. The first popular "high-protein" diet book was published in 1864 by an English casket maker named William Banting.

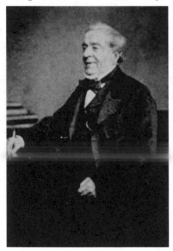 During this same era, P.T. Barnum told Americans "There's a sucker born every minute," and the casket-maker's diet did, among other things, prove P.T. Barnum right. The Atkins Diet, Zone Diet, South Beach and other "high-protein" diets all have their roots in, appropriately enough, a casket maker's diet because they all contribute to heart disease, kidney disease, osteoporosis and our common cancers, not to mention the constipation, gastrointestinal difficulties, bad breath and other symptoms that are the result of "high protein" diets. Little wonder the American Dietetic Association has described these diets as "a nightmare." The phrase "high-protein" is simply a euphemism for "high-fat" to disguise the fact these diets are plowing an incredibly unhealthy diet down your throat, with the Atkins Diet being up to 60 percent fat.

The fact that Banting's diet was all the rage in the late 1800's and Atkins-like diets are now the rage over 100 years later shows: 1) how little progress we have made in making people understand such quick fixes don't work; 2) the power of advertising; and 3) how such diets come into vogue when the price of meat is cheap. People think Atkins has come up with something new in the diet field. All he did was popularize a failed diet that was over 100 years old.

---

[13] Foryet, J. Limitations of behavioral treatment of obesity: review and analysis. 1981, J. Behav. Med. 4:159-73.

Now, take a deep breath because I want you to think about something. Don't you think it's strange – perhaps more than a little embarrassing – that none of these diet plans work in the long term, yet we keep shelling out money only to prove that history does repeat itself – at least when it comes to diet plans? Have Americans become so desperate that common sense has totally gone out the window?

Think about it. We're in such pathetic shape that the most educated population on the face of the earth now needs a doctor to tell them how to eat. In the meantime, billions of "uneducated" people throughout the world are in better health than most Americans, keep slim figures and many have never even seen a doctor. It's only a slight exaggeration to say that people were getting better advice about what they should eat when they were seeing witch doctors.

The goal of weight loss is to reduce the percentage of body fat and you cannot lose body fat quickly. Any program that promises quick weight loss is not losing fat, but simply water. Losing weight is not complicated at all. In fact, it's quite simple and the Diet Doctors have done more to confuse the issue than anyone else. (See *Notes - Problems With the Glycemic Index*, for one example.) But there's a method to their madness: The more complicated dieting seems, the more money there is to be made from all the confusion. And although these diets don't work – even for the Diet Doctors – the good doctors are more than willing to accept your money for the advice they're selling, advice they can't even follow themselves.

Why are things so insane? In a word: money. Selling food, supplements and diet plans is big money. Selling the easy way out is big money. Telling people they can lose more weight watching TV than exercising is big money.

Once all the fog has lifted, you'll see just how simple it is to lose weight. You won't have to buy expensive supplements or special foods, join programs, make yourself miserable or participate in any of the money-making schemes designed to impoverish you. Americans are now spending over $40 billion dollars a year in their desperate efforts to shed pounds and get thin. What diet ads should say is "I lost $350 in two week! Ask me how!" And the vast majority of these bucks flow into the pockets of people with an M.D. or Ph.D. behind their names – and most should be ashamed of themselves for not telling people the truth about weight loss, but instead perpetuating a self-enrichment scam.

Weight loss involves much more than counting calories and eating the right foods. Losing weight is not about the body – it's about the mind. It's about changing the way you think about food. It's also about changing the way you think about life. Your weight is the most visible reflection of who you are and losing weight involves nothing short of fundamentally changing your life. Change your life first, then the weight will come off naturally – and stay off.

We all know the story of the tortoise and the hare. Popular diets are about the hare that loses weight very fast, but ends up losing the race because the pounds return over time. The tortoise, on the other hand, is slow but steady and ends up winning the race by losing weight slowly and surely – and keeping it off for a lifetime.

The RAVE Diet & Lifestyle is a long-term health regimen designed not only to lose weight, but also to enhance your health and energy level and to prevent (and even reverse) the common diseases that are ravaging Americans today. Most diet plans start with a bang and have you lose 20 pounds in a few months. I would rather you change your eating habits first and gradually lose those 20 pounds over the course of a year so they will stay off the rest of your life and never come back.

If you're reading this book because you've tried the Diet Doctors and failed, take heart because the road to success is usually paved with failure. I believe that knowledge is power. Just as a good stockbroker uses his knowledge of stocks to make you a profit, knowledge of food will make you thin and give you all the benefits that come with such a lifestyle.

Being overweight affects all aspects of your life and it becomes cumulative. Your self-respect declines, you stay in more, you become more sedentary, you eat for comfort and end up putting on even more weight. If you're going to achieve success in weight loss, you are going to have to take an honest look at yourself, what you're eating and how you're living. The purpose of this book is to help you do just that.

We're in a state of denial about our weight and as our waistlines expand, we've lost sight of what normal weight is. We keep growing bigger and bigger

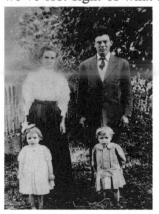

and think it's normal because we've become used to it. Unfortunately, what's normal to Americans in the 21st century is fat. Have you ever looked at those old-time pictures of working-class people living in the 1800s from a weight perspective? Then compare their bodies to ours now? The only fat people you will see in those old pictures are wealthy people, who could afford to eat much like Americans eat today. The average working-class American back in those times was thin because they were doing two things correctly: eating the right foods and getting exercise.

Being overweight – and especially being obese – can lead to a host of diseases, among them heart disease. The only scientifically proven diets to reverse heart disease are RAVE Diets. In fact, the RAVE Diet is a friendlier version of other diets that are used to reverse heart disease. No other diet can show actual proof of heart disease reversal. None. And if you eat to prevent heart disease, you will prevent the other major chronic diseases that are plaguing Western nations, including diabetes, our common cancers, as well as hundreds of other diet-related diseases.

In other words, you will get much, much more out of the RAVE Diet than just permanent weight loss. You'll get a lifetime of good health.

Diet, Disease & Weight Loss

"Most people don't let their children smoke, yet they regularly take them to fast-food restaurants and that's just as risky, in terms of cancer, as if they had bought them a pack of Marlborough cigarettes." – B. A. Stoll

"There is only one major disease and that is malnutrition. All ailments and afflictions to which we may fall heir are directly traceable to this major disease." – D.W. Cavanaugh, M.D., Cornell University

There is an old Indian legend in which six blind men come across an elephant. Having no idea what an elephant was, they moved in close and started to feel it.

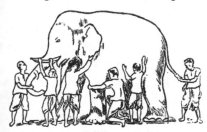

One touched its leg and described the elephant as a pillar. Another touched its tail and declared an elephant was a rope. The third touched its ear and said the elephant was like a big fan. And so on. The blind men then began to argue about what an elephant was, based on the empirical data they had collected – with each insisting he was correct. The problem, of course, was that none of the blind men could "see" the entire elephant, only parts of it.

Many of the problems that Americans have with understanding the relationship of diet to disease are analogous to this story. Unfortunately, the inability to see the whole picture is greatly reinforced by so-called "scientific" studies because they only look at specific parts of the entire picture.

Take alcoholic beverages, for example. Recently, there have been waves of studies purporting that wine is good for the heart. This is because these studies are focusing only on a small part of the wine, the antioxidants, which originally came from grapes. What such studies cannot "see" is the alcohol in the wine. When you step back and look at the whole wine beverage, including alcohol, wine not only harms the heart, but the brain, nervous system, liver and other organs – and generally devastates the entire body. Instead of saying that wine is good for the heart and ignoring what it does to the rest of the body, the "scientists" should have been saying this study confirms that the antioxidants found in grapes are good for the heart, without endorsing wine as a health beverage.[1]

---

[1] The latest round of silly studies reveals that wine is not only good for the heart, but it will prevent physical disabilities, fights Alzheimer's, boosts Omega 3 levels, and lowers

We have known that antioxidants are good for the heart for decades. And we have known that grapes are good for the body for centuries. What such "scientific" studies are doing is turning bad foods into good foods for the sole benefit of those who sell bad foods. (Don't get me wrong. If you want to get tipsy or even drunk, there's no better beverage than wine – just don't call it a health drink!)

Of course, the "scientific" approach fits very nicely into the marketing plans of food industries and, in fact, virtually all of these "scientific" studies are funded by food industries. These days, if a product has even a tiny bit of good in it, food industries will hire a team of "experts" from a prestigious university to do a study specifically designed to turn an unhealthy product into a "healthy" product. They will then put out press releases and unleash their marketing team to "milk" as much news coverage from the study as they can get. The public then reads the news report and thinks, "Ah ha! Wine is good for me, after all!" and they run to the nearest liquor store and start drinking like fish.

After a "60 Minutes" show ran a story on the so-called French Paradox, which made the ridiculous claim that wine was responsible for the deceptively low rate of heart attacks in France, wine sales increased by a whopping 40 percent. What was lost in all the hoopla was the fact that the French Paradox is a mirage. The French have different methods of classifying deaths, which make it appear that deaths due to heart disease are lower in France than other Western nations. When statistical methods are standardized, however, it turns out the French die of heart disease at rates comparable to other Western nations. And regardless of how you view the statistics, heart disease is France's number one killer, just as it is in other Western nations who eat comparable diets.[2]

The dairy industry is famous for sponsoring "scientific" studies showing the benefits of consuming their products due to the calcium content. And because the dairy lobby has many politicians in their pocket, our official calcium requirements are now absurdly high. Surprisingly, no one has ever thought to ask why we need ever-higher amounts of calcium in our diet when there has never been a single recorded instance of calcium deficiency of a dietary origin in the history of the human race![3]

---

lung cancer risks! All of which, of course, is ultimately good for the wine industry. "Four More Reasons to Drink Red Wine," Newsweek, 1/23/09.

[2] Eat Right, Live Longer, Neal Barnard, M.D., p. 35.

[3] There are all kinds of bone diseases, e.g., rickets, but none is the result of a dietary deficiency of calcium. In other words, any natural diet will provide enough calcium for the human body. Calcium Requirements in man: a critical review, C. Paterson, Postgrad Med J. 54:244, 1978; The human requirement of calcium: should low intakes be supplemented? A. Walker, Am J. Clin Nutr, 25:518, 1972; Symposium on human calcium requirements: Council on Foods and Nutrition, JAMA 185:588, 1963; Modern Nutrition in Health and Disease, 5th ed, Goodhart and Shils, 1973, p. 274.

Despite this fact, the dairy industry – backed by the authority of the USDA – has scared the wits out of women who think the calcium in dairy products will somehow magically bind to their bones, make them strong and prevent osteoporosis. (See *Notes - Osteoporosis* for more on this subject.)

What the dairy industry does is simply hire a bunch of blind scientists and instructs them to focus on a single ingredient in order to turn an incredibly bad food (high levels of sodium, cholesterol, saturated fat and animal protein) into a good food. Recently, they funded a study which made the ridiculous claim that calcium was the key to losing weight![4]

We could go down the list of so-called scientific studies which purport to show the benefits of a single ingredient in a food (e.g., the "good fat" in vegetable oils, the "good fat" in fish, flavonoids in chocolate candy bars), while ignoring the package of bad ingredients these good ingredients come in. These studies, of course, are nothing but marketing tools employed by food industries working on a gullible public trying their best to find a healthy meal somewhere in America.

In the meantime, Americans get sicker from eating bad foods the scientific community has declared "healthy." Of course, the sicker they get from eating bad foods, the more it feeds into a bottom-feeder – the pharmaceutical industry. In an effort to counteract a bad diet, we end up taking medicines to treat symptoms of diseases that are the result of eating bad foods – primarily because a bunch of functionally blind scientists told us these bad foods were good for us.

During the 1800s, there was a doctor who followed the medically approved bleeding and drugging procedures of the time, but eventually lost confidence in these procedures because he saw that the health of his patients was not improving. In fact, he found that his patients started to get much better when he prescribed fewer or no drugs. Following a hunch, he decided to eliminate the drugs and bleedings altogether and give patients placebos, or sugar pills, instead. At the same time he gave them advice about improving their diet.

The key to this approach was that he told his patients *the pill would not work unless they followed the diet he prescribed.* Well, his patients followed his dietary advice to the letter, thinking the pill would not work unless they followed the diet, and much to their surprise, the "pill" worked! The diseases in his patients quickly vanished and the good doctor's fame spread rapidly. He soon became known as the greatest healer of his time – for all the wrong reasons. No one talked about the diet he prescribed and all his patients could do was blather about his wonderful magic pills.[5]

It's been estimated that 70 to 85 percent of all hospital patients suffer from illnesses associated with diet-induced diseases.[6] This should not come as a

---

[4] Calcium could be key to weight loss, The Seattle Times, 4/21/04.
[5] Fasting and Eating for Health, Joel Fuhrman, M.D., p. 56.
[6] Caldwell B. Esselstyn, M.D., as stated in the film Eating by Mike Anderson, The McDougall Program, John A. McDougall, M.D., p. 17.

surprise. Throughout history, humans have lived primarily on a diet of whole, natural plant foods. Today, whole plant foods constitute *only seven percent of our diet!* Forty-two percent of our calories come from animal foods and a whopping 51 percent of our calories come from refined foods.[7]

Historical Percent of Total Calories

Animal foods	5 percent [8]
Refined foods	0 percent
Whole plant foods	<u>95 percent</u>

Current Percent of Total Calories

Animal foods	42 percent
Refined foods	51 percent
Whole plant foods	<u>7 percent</u>

In other words, animal and refined foods – which contain neither fiber nor cancer-fighting or heart-healthy nutrients – make up a whopping 93 percent of the calories we consume today. It doesn't take much imagination to see how our diet is driving us into hospitals.

During the long history of humans, we ate 95 percent of our calories from whole plant foods. The precipitous fall in whole plant food consumption began only a century ago.

It should be obvious that disease would follow our switch from a plant-based to an animal- and refined-foods-based diet and this accounts for the explosion of the chronic, degenerative diseases and common cancers which are currently affecting every family in America today. Below is a brief summary of the differences between plant foods, animal and refined foods.

---

[7] Eat To Live, Joel Fuhrman, M.D., p. 51. In this estimate, oils constitute 11% of total calories. Oils are considered a refined food.

[8] Estimates vary somewhat, depending on the authority, but according to world-renowned paleontologist Dr. Richard Leakey, animal foods were a very rare part of the human evolutionary diet. The five percent used here is hypothetical and may be lower. [Dr. Richard Leakey, as quoted in The Power of Your Plate, Neal Barnard, M.D., p. 170.] When ancient man did eat meat, he probably walked, ran and jumped 20 miles to get it. And, aside from a very few areas where meat was plentiful, ancient man ate meat only a few times a year. In addition, the composition of wild game was a far cry from our grain-fed, domesticated, high-fat, hormone-laced meat that almost all Americans eat today. There were, of course, some populations late in our history that ate higher amounts of meat. They did, however, suffer the consequences. Autopsy studies of meat-eating specimens, such as the Iceman, have shown advanced stages of heart disease in 25 year olds.

Whole Plant Foods	Animal Foods	Refined Foods
Fiber	No Fiber	No Fiber
Cancer fighters	No cancer fighters	No cancer fighters
Anti-oxidants	Oxidants	Oxidants
Low fat	High fat	High fat
Low saturated fat	High saturated fat	High saturated fat
No cholesterol	High cholesterol	High trans fat
Low pesticides/toxins	High pesticides/toxins [9]	High sugar
No hormones	High hormones [10]	

The Magic of Whole Plant Foods

The best, simplest and most cost-effective way Americans can vastly improve their health and prevent our major diseases is to radically increase their consumption of whole, natural plant foods. Unlike foods that may have a single "good" nutrient that comes in a package of bad nutrients, whole natural foods do not have such tradeoffs. Whole foods are good for the whole body. They are not just "heart-healthy," they are healthy for the heart, the brain, the arteries and all organs. They are "entire" body-healthy.

How good are whole foods? We are just at the beginning of our understanding. Let me give you an illustration. In the 1970s, there was a study conducted in

---

[9] It's been estimated that meat and dairy foods account for over 90 percent of the population's intake of pesticides. This is due to the heavy pesticide use on crops destined for consumption by farm animals. Far lower levels of pesticides are used on crops destined for human consumption. These pesticide-laden crops are fed to farm animals and they end up in the tissues and fat that we eat. The higher on the food chain you eat, the more concentrated the pesticides.

[10] The use of hormones in cattle is so great that Europe has banned American beef from its shores. Stephany, R.W., Hormones in meat: Different approaches in the EU and in the USA, APMIS 109:S357. And dairy is essentially a hormonal factory, containing dozens of active hormones to fuel the growth of a calf that will weigh up to 500 pounds within a year of its birth. Here are some of them: Pituitary hormones (PRL, GH, TSH, FSH, LH ACTH Oxytocin); Steroid hormones (Estradiol, Estriol, Progesterone, Testosterone, 17-Ketosteroids, Corticosterone, Vitamine D); Hypothalamic hormones (TRH, LHRH, Somatostatin, PRL-inhibiting factor, PRL-releasing factor, GnRH, GRH); Thyroid and Parathyroid hormones (T3, T4, rT3, Calcitonin, Parathormone, PTH peptide); gastrointestinal peptides (Vasoactive intestinal peptide, Bombesin, Cholecystokinin, Gastrin, Gastrin inhibitory peptide, Pancreatic peptide, Y peptide, Substance P and Neurotensin); Growth Factors (IGF's (I and II), IGF binding proteins, Nerve growth factor, Epidermal growth factor and TGF alpha, TGF beta, Growth Inhibitors MDGI and MAF, and Platelet derived growth factor; Others... (PGE, PGF2 alpha, cAMP, cGMP, Delta sleep inducing peptide, Transferrin, Lactoferrin, Casomorphin and Erythropoietin.

which animals were fed two percent of their diet from red dye, sodium cyclamate or an emulsifier. The animals that were fed just one additive showed no harmful effects at all. The animals that were fed two of the additives showed balding fur, diarrhea and retarded weight gain. But the animals that were fed all three additives were dead within two weeks.[11]

In a similar fashion, it was recently reported that Parkinson's disease has been linked to the exposure of not one, but a combination of pesticides, namely paraquat and organophosphate.[12]

What this illustrates is that toxins, when taken together, *amplify* their toxicity in a synergistic and logarithmic fashion.

In a similar – but beneficial – way, nutrients work together in the same way, e.g., calcium with magnesium, vitamin E with selenium, protein with B6 and so forth. There are also thousands of antioxidants that work together in a synergistic fashion which multiplies their health-enhancing effects. A tomato, for example, contains over 10,000 different phytochemicals. The possible combinations and permutations of nutrients once inside the body are simply mind-boggling. And, at this point, we have only a child-like understanding of how these nutrients work together in literally hundreds of thousands of combinations.

There have been a number of studies that show when a single chemo-preventive nutrient is fed to animals it had no effect on the incidence of cancer. But when two or more nutrients were combined, the cancer growth was sharply cut.[13] What these studies examined was just a few nutrients, not the thousands and thousands of combinations that go on inside your body every day in the real world.

Remember when vitamin C was the rage? Everyone was taking vitamin C tablets like they were going out of style. Then it was discovered that vitamin C wasn't very well absorbed unless a couple of bioflavonoids were present (hesperidin and rutin). So the manufacturers re-tooled and added these bioflavonoids to the pills and everything was supposed to be Ok again. Except it was later discovered that despite the presence of these bioflavonoids, the body couldn't absorb vitamin C very well unless calcium was present, as well. So the pills were re-formulated with bioflavonoids *and* calcium. So, while the public remained confused – but nonetheless kept swallowing their vitamin C tablets – they continued to overlook a source of vitamin C that had *all* the elements together and allowed optimal absorption of the vitamin: citrus fruits, such as oranges and grapefruits – as well as a myriad of other plant foods bearing vitamin C! While "blind" scientists were baffled trying to come up with one or two or three key ingredients that would allow the body to effectively absorb vitamin C

---

[11] These additives were all FDA approved at the time. Ershoff, BH, J. of Food Science, vol. 41, p. 949, 1976.

[12] New Study Suggests Chemicals Could Trigger Disease, AP, 11/6/00.

[13] Japanese J. Cancer Research, Rao, AR, et al., vol. 81, p. 1239.

in pill form, people forgot that nature had already come up with a solution to this problem in the form of whole plant foods, which contain thousands of nutrient profiles scientists are still in the dark about.[14]

The point is this: When scientists try to isolate a single nutrient or even a handful of nutrients, this is not only overly simplistic, but also doomed to misleading results and failure. In fact, this kind of analysis is like the six blind men trying to understand the nature of an elephant. While science will continue to identify key nutrients in foods, it is a certainty that science will never understand how the millions of nutrients interact with each other. The mathematical possibilities are simply too immense.

When I say there is "magic" in whole foods, I'm talking about what we do not understand about whole foods – and that is far more than we do know.   What we *do* know, however, is that they are good for us – in fact, far and away much better for us than anything ever created by science. What we do know is that we should eat a wide variety of foods because each food has its own nutrient profile and this profile will interact with other foods containing their own profile and together, they will multiply, in logarithmic fashion, each other's protective benefits.

When a diet is practically devoid of whole plant foods, only trouble can result. In such a situation, Americans are turning to supplements in order to bolster an inadequate diet – but supplements cannot possibly replace the potency of whole foods containing a multitude of nutrient profiles we haven't even a clue about. In every study ever conducted which compared supplements with whole plant foods, supplements could not hold a candle to the power and potency of whole foods. A recent study showed that taking supplements, containing lycopene from tomatoes, did *nothing* to lower the risk of prostate cancer, whereas whole tomatoes, containing a complex profile of nutrients, did lower the risk.[15] How it lowered the risk, scientists haven't a clue because nature is far too complex to be understood with our crude tools. And, once again, this illustrates the failure of trying to isolate a single nutrient as a cure to a disease and sell it to the public as a "magic bullet."

The bottom line is that no matter how hard they try, scientists cannot capture the "magical" nutrient profiles of whole foods in a pill and that magic can only be passed into your body by eating them.

---

[14] Lessons From the Miracle Doctors, Jon Barron, p. 54
[15] Tomatoes May Be Better Against Cancer Than Lycopene Alone, LA Times, 11/10/03.

A Diet of Disease

No matter how strange something is, if you give it enough time, it becomes normal. Americans have now accepted heart disease, cancer and other degenerative diseases as a normal part of the American way of life.

One could not design a diet more efficient at clogging arteries than the American diet. Between animal foods and refined foods, our arteries don't have a chance. What amazes me is that everyone doesn't die of heart disease.

The war on cancer does not take place in hospitals or laboratories. It takes place inside you and battles are being won or lost every day, depending on your diet.

"Each patient carries his own doctor inside him. We are at our best when we give the doctor who resides within a chance to go to work." Albert Schweitzer, Nobel Prize Winner

The Laws of Heart Disease

Before 1900, heart disease was virtually unknown and so rare it wasn't even included in standard American medical textbooks.[16] Today, heart disease (cardiovascular disease) is the scourge of the nation. Practically everyone has heart disease, children are now taking heart medicines, and it's the biggest killer in the nation – killing more than half the population – yet it's the single most preventable major disease there is. Heart disease has become so prevalent that drug makers are now working to make cholesterol-lowering drugs non-prescription so taking them will be as easy as taking an aspirin. They've already made it that way in Britain.

While everyone is concentrating their efforts on selling drugs that *treat* heart disease, very few are talking about *curing* the disease. And almost everyone ignores the fact that a disease that kills over half the population and maims even more is solely the result of a bad diet.

And yet, heart disease can be easily cured with a change to the RAVE Diet. Heart disease isn't just preventable – it's *reversible*, no matter what your age. Heart disease immediately responds to changes in diet, as the body begins to heal itself once the onslaught of bad foods stops.

According to William Castelli, director of the famous Framingham Heart Study, entire populations have reversed heart disease by changing their diet.

---

[16] Eat To Beat Cancer, J. Robert Hatherhill, p. 17, 50. Note: most people died of infectious diseases, not degenerative diseases.

Before World War II, about three-quarters of the people in Belgium suffered from heart disease. During the German occupation, however, soldiers trucked every scrap of meat and all the livestock out of Belgium to Germany. Within two years, their rates of heart disease and cancer plummeted in the Belgium population, *because they had no meat to eat*. These diseases also vanished from the landscape in every other country where Germany removed livestock, including Holland, Poland and Norway, as well as northern France. Unfortunately, as farm animals returned to these countries after the war, so too did heart disease.[17]

Incredulous as it may seem, advocates of high-fat diets will argue that meat-based diets can prevent and even reverse heart disease. The problem with such an argument is that there has never been a single human being who has ever arrested or reversed heart disease on meat-based diets.

Reversing heart disease is actually a very simple and inexpensive thing to do and there are literally millions of Americans dying to have their heart disease reversed on meat-based diets. Since there are so many people on "high-protein" diets, one would think that out of those millions, just one person would have reversed his or her heart disease – even by accident!

You have to ask yourself, "Why haven't the high-protein people recruited someone with severe heart disease and reversed it?" If they had just a single individual who reversed heart disease on their diet, he or she would become the poster boy for that diet overnight – and their publicity machine would have a field day. Why hasn't this been done? It would only take six months and they would have publicity to last them years. Then everyone could eat steak and eggs for breakfast.

I say to these people, stop the arguments and stop citing so-called "scientific" studies. Show me a real human being who has reversed heart disease on anything other than a RAVE Diet.

Long silence.

In fact, no one has ever arrested or reversed heart disease on anything but a RAVE Diet.

Of course, trans-fats or hydrogenated oils can also be a cause of heart disease. Those who promote high-fat diets have seized on this fact and cite trans-fats as the main cause of heart disease. This argument not only ignores clinical studies and over 50 years of solid medical research, but also ignores common sense. When cows are fed meat, for example, they develop heart disease – just like we do – and no cow that I know of has ever eaten an Oreo cookie. Similarly, autopsies of prehistoric humans who ate meat-heavy diets in certain areas of the world have shown heart disease in 25-year-olds. And to my knowledge, they never had Krispe Kreme donuts for breakfast while sitting around the campfire.

---

[17] The Power of Your Plate, Neal Barnard, M.D., p. 23; A Solution to the Cancer Problem, Cornelius. Moerman, M.D., p. 31.

There are also cases where people have actually reversed heart disease following a RAVE Diet, but then returned to eating meat – and their heart disease returned, as well. When an animal-based diet is introduced to populations, which never had heart disease in their history, heart disease becomes their number one killer. And when meat is taken away from populations, such as those cited above during World War II, heart disease is reversed.

To blame this disease on trans-fats, while saying it's Ok to eat high levels of saturated fat and cholesterol, high-fat advocates are providing people with very dangerous advice. It simply boils down to yet another diversionary tactic in order to keep people on meat-based diets – and keep the revenues of high-fat diet programs fat.

Another related argument of the high-fat set is that during the last 20 years, Americans were eating *less* fat, yet getting fatter, so lowering dietary fat doesn't result in weight loss. The conclusion: It isn't the fat that's making us fat, but the carbs. So follow a low-carb diet! As appealing as this argument may seem, it is completely false. In fact, Americans are now eating more fat than ever. The basic problem is that they are also eating more *calories* than ever. As a result, the *percentage of fat* from total calories has declined, but the total fat in our diet has actually *increased.*[18]

The arguments of the high-fat priesthood are not only lame and deceptive, but there are also big differences in honesty between high-fat and low-fat advocates, as illustrated in how the deaths of Dr. Nathan Pritikin and Dr. Robert Atkins were handled. Pritikin, who followed a RAVE Diet when he reversed his own heart disease, stipulated in his will that he should be autopsied and the results published, regardless of the outcome. Following his will's directives, his body was autopsied and it was found he had the heart and arteries of a young man, which were completely clear of any signs of heart disease or atherosclerosis. He had, indeed, totally reversed his heart disease with diet and the results of his autopsy were published in the New England Journal of Medicine.[19]

In stark contrast, everything possible was done to conceal the health of Dr. Atkins before and after his death, despite claims by the Atkins people his diet was "heart-healthy" and despite decades of solid medical research showing such a diet to be stupendously heart un-healthy. In fact, a recent study has shown that the Atkins diet reduces blood flow to the heart by 40 percent after just one year.[20]

High amounts of any kind of fat, be it vegetable fats or animal fats, decrease the amount of oxygen delivery to the body. After a high-fat meal, doctors can actually see blood sludging in the whites of patients' eyes, due to the high

---

[18] J Am Diet Assoc. 2003 Jul;103(7):867-72.

[19] New England Journal of Medicine, July 4, 1985.

[20] The effect of high-protein diets on coronary blood flow, Fleming RM, Angiology 2000;51(10):817-826.

concentration of fat.[21] A blood sample taken from a man a few hours after eating a cheeseburger and shake revealed that *half* of the blood sample consisted of fat.[22] American blood is so thick with fat that doctors are now scrambling to put millions of patients on aspirin therapy in an effort just to thin their blood.

Some people try to justify a 30 percent fat diet by pleading we *need* lots of fat in our diet. But, in fact, the amount of fat you *need* is tiny – just 3 to 4 percent of total calories from fat.[23] In other words, a 30 percent fat diet (what mainstream medicine calls a low-fat diet) is giving you 10 times the amount of fat that you actually need – and most Americans eat a 40 percent plus fat diet. In fact, there has never been a recorded case of fat deficiency of a dietary origin in the history of mankind. Even prisoners of war do not suffer from too little fat in their diets! That Americans should worry about getting enough fat is a sad commentary on how we've been hoodwinked by high-fat food industries and the U.S. government that supports them.

With respect to heart disease, there are two "laws" that are, to date, irrefutable.

1) Heart disease can only be reversed on a true low-fat diet (10% or less of total calories).
2) Heart attacks do not occur with people having total cholesterol levels under 150.

The RAVE Diet will show you how to achieve a 10 percent fat level with delicious foods so you can reverse heart disease – and if you eat to prevent or reverse heart disease, you'll be preventing all the other degenerative diseases that are making Americans sick and causing them to die prematurely. That is the ticket the RAVE Diet has for you on the health train.

On a heart disease prevention diet – as opposed to a reversal diet – the maximum fat level is 20 percent of total calories. Since most adult Americans already have heart disease, you should try to reverse it as much as possible by getting your fat level down to 10 percent by strictly following the RAVE Diet.

While medical authorities are fiddling with LDL and HDL levels and ratios, your goal should not be a ratio, but a total cholesterol level below 150. If you do that, you'll never have to worry about having a heart attack again. And you

---

[21] Serum lipids and conjunctival circulation after fat ingestion in men exhibiting type-A behavior pattern, Friedman, M., Circulation 29:874, 1964 ; Effect of unsaturated fats upon lipemia and conjunctival circulation. A study of coronary-prone (pattern A) men., Friedman, M., JAMA 193: 882, 1965; John A. McDougall, M.D., A Challenging Second Opinion, p. 157. Citation: The effect of lipemia upon coronary and peripheral arterial circulation in patients with essential hyperlipemia, Juo, P., Amer J Med 26:68, 1959 Re 40% Fleming RM. The effect of high-protein diets on coronary blood flow. Angiology 2000;51(10):817-826.

[22] As shown in the film, *Eating*. www.RaveDiet.com.

[23] Breaking the Food Seduction, Neal Barnard, M.D., 160.

simply cannot get your cholesterol level below 150 unless you adopt a RAVE Diet.[24]

People like to scoff at the idea that diet is so powerful, preferring to take expensive medicines instead. They will point to studies that show a change in fat levels does not have an effect on diseases. The problem with these studies is that they make small dietary changes. For example, they may reduce a 40 percent fat diet to a 30 percent fat diet and say the dietary fat level does not make a difference. That's like switching from regular cigarettes to light cigarettes and that won't prevent anything.

What you have to do is make a *big* change before you'll be able to reverse and prevent our diet-related diseases. What medical authorities have to do is reduce dietary fat from 40 percent to 10 percent before they will see a difference – and it will be a *huge* difference. It's also been shown that a diet of 10 percent fat is far more effective than heart disease medicines in lowering LDL cholesterol levels – and diet does not have any side effects.[25]

Following mainstream advice to eat more fruits and vegetables simply will not get the job done. It's a bit like adding a couple of raisins to a chocolate bar and declaring that chocolate bar to be healthy. In order to realize the healing effects of plant foods, you have to make a complete switch and do it in an uncompromising fashion. The RAVE Diet & Lifestyle shows you how to do just that.

The Laws of Cancer

"During the past fifty years scientists experimenting with thousands of animals have found 700 ways of causing cancer. But they had not discovered one way of curing the disease." – J. F. Brailsford, M.D.

We have spent over 30 years and countless billions of tax dollars trying to find a cure for cancer, yet Nature has been solving the dilemma from the beginning. The cure for cancer is right inside all of us. It's called your immune system.

Your immune system is your internal body armor. Picture your immune system as the front defensive line of a football team. The mission of this defensive line (your white blood cells) is to stop the other team (cancer cells) from getting through and scoring points. If the defensive line, your immune system, is weak or injured the other team gets through causing damage and

---

[24] Due to genetics, there is a small percentage of the population that can achieve total cholesterol levels below 150, regardless of their diet.

[25] Barnard ND, Scialli AR, Bertron P, et al. Effectiveness of a low-fat vegetarian diet in altering serum lipids in healthy premenopausal women. Am J Cardiol 2000 Apr 15;85(8):969-72.

scoring points. How do you build up your defensive team? The *only* way is through diet.

For years Japan had the highest per capita consumption of cigarettes, yet the lowest rates of lung cancer in the world, because Japanese smokers had strong immune systems due to their low-fat, plant-based diet.[26] Of course, now that the Japanese diet is becoming westernized, they are compromising their immune systems and cancer is on the rise. Cancer is scoring points.

With respect to cancer, there are four "laws" that are irrefutable.

1) Your immune system is the only cure for cancer.
2) A weakened immune system is the biggest cause of cancer.[27]
3) The higher the dietary fat, the more the immune system is weakened.
4) The only foods that contain immune-strengthening and cancer-fighting nutrients are plant foods.

Your eating habits can either strengthen or weaken your immune system. If you are not eating enough plant foods, you will be deficient in the antioxidants and phytochemicals that feed an army of immune system cells that defend the body against cancer. Your immune system has been trained over millions of years to recognize and selectively kill cancer cells and is at least a million times smarter at killing them than sledge-hammer-like conventional treatments, such as

---

[26] Eat To Beat Cancer, J. Robert Hatherhill, p. 59. Of course, this hardly implies the Japanese have an ideal diet. Their high rates of stomach cancer have been blamed on the high sodium content of their diet. Corroborating evidence has recently been gathered by studies showing vegetable intake reduces the risks of smoking-related cancers. Veg-eating smokers 'cheat illness': Increasing fruit intake may boost your chances," BBC News, 7/31/02; "Veggies cut smokers' cancer risk," MSNBC, 4/8/02; Protective effects of raw vegetables and fruit against lung cancer among smokers and ex-smokers: a case-control study in the Tokai area of Japan, C.M. Gao, K. Tajima, T. Kuroishi, et al, 1993, Japan J. Cancer Res. 84 (6): 594-600.

[27] Genetics accounts for only a small percentage of our common cancers. In the case of breast cancer, for example, genetics accounts for only 5% of all cases. In terms of other external factors, air and water pollution only account for 5%, alcohol and radiation account for 3% each, and medications account for only 2% of cancers. Tobacco use accounts for 30% and the balance is due to dietary factors. For many individuals, genetics may make a contribution in subtle ways, e.g., it may determine one's susceptibility to carcinogens, the strength of the immune system, body weight, and other factors. But each of these is also influenced by diet and such weaknesses can be offset by dietary habits, as illustrated in the Japanese smoker example. For more discussion on this topic, see *Notes - Genetics*, Notes. Sources: Minamoto T, Mai M, Ronai Z. Environmental factors as regulators and effectors of multistep carcinogenesis. Carcinogenesis 1999;20(4):519-27; Cummings JH, Bingham SA. Diet and the prevention of cancer. BMJ 1998;317:1636-40.

chemotherapy or radiation. Those treatments indiscriminately kill cancer cells while also killing the only cure for cancer – your immune system cells.

In every population throughout the world eating an animal-based diet, cancer is the second leading killer, after heart disease. Among other things, due to the high-fat content, animal-based diets suppress the immune system by killing off immune system cells.

Imagine what an oil spill in the ocean does to the marine life it encounters. Most are killed, some are maimed. Birds covered with oil cannot fly. This is what happens when high amounts of fat hit your blood stream. Immune system cells die off, those that survive cannot "swim" in your blood stream, they become blinded and as a result cannot recognize and kill cancer cells. Now imagine eating three high-fat meals a day. Americans have created a constant oil slick in their blood streams, which is caused by breakfast, lunch and dinner.

The higher your intake of fat, the more your immune system is weakened, which leaves you open to infections and diseases. We have an epidemic of immune system impairment and this accounts for many of the diseases we are suffering from, especially cancers. In fact, we've become so used to a suppressed immune system that we now think it's normal. We also think that dying of cancer is a normal part of the human condition. It is not.

Any kind of fat will compromise the immune system, even so-called "good fats" containing Omega-3 fatty acids. In addition to being an oil slick, it's been found that Omega-3's that come in concentrated forms, such as fish and vegetable oils, are composed of highly unstable molecules which decompose and unleash dangerous cancer-causing agents (free radicals), and cause damage to cells that can lead to cancer. Such fats also suppress natural killer cells and the production of immune substances, which are important not only for cancer protection, but protection against viruses, bacteria and parasites.[28]

High concentrations of Omega-3's also promote the *spread* of cancer cells. This is thought to be due to the production of free radicals, suppression of the immune system and changes that are caused in small hormones that promote tumor growth.[29]

Unlike concentrated fats in fish and vegetable oils, the Omega-3s found in natural, whole foods are *stable* and do not produce free radicals. Thus, if you want Omega-3s, get them from whole plant foods, not vegetable or fish oils.

---

[28] Health implications of the n-3 fatty acids, Odeleye OE, Watson RR., Am J Clin Nutr 1991;53:177-8; Reply to O Odeleye and R Watson, Kinsella JE, Am J Clin Nutr 1991;53:178.

[29] Effects of fish oil and corn oil diets on prostaglandin-dependent and myelopoiesis-associated immune suppressor mechanisms of mice bearing metastatic Lewis lung carcinoma tumors, Young MR, Cancer Res. 1989 Apr 15;49(8):1931-6; Influence of lipid diets on the number of metastases and ganglioside content of H59 variant tumors, Coulombe J, Clin Exp Metastasis. 1997 Jul;15(4):410-7.

Eating concentrated sources of "good fat" really boils down to getting too much of a good thing. Just as a modest amount of sunlight can actually prevent cancer,[30] too much sunlight can cause cancer. Just as we need a little saturated fat in our diet, too much can clog up our plumbing. When vegetable oils are made, thousands of nutrients, as well as the fiber, are removed and all that's left is 100 percent fat, or empty calories. This is an extremely concentrated form of fat and too much of a good thing, which will cause bad things to happen, like an oil slick in your blood. (For more on vegetable oils, see *The RAVE Diet & Lifestyle: No Vegetable Oils*.)

The high-fat content of animal-based foods significantly suppresses the immune system, so it's little wonder that heart disease and cancer are America's two biggest killers. Lowering the fat in your diet is not only the best thing for your heart, but it's also the single best way to strengthen your immune system. Instead of a steady stream of fat, the RAVE Diet will lower your fat intake and give you a steady stream of cancer-fighting nutrients that will feed your immune system and keep it strong.

Hormonal Cancers: Breast and Prostate

Excessive dietary fat not only suppresses the immune system, but it also stimulates the abnormally high production sex hormones, which greatly increases the risk of developing hormone-related cancers, such as breast and prostate cancer. Any time you take a bite into a hamburger, hot dog, chicken leg or any other high-fat meal, you're not only weakening your immune system, but you're getting a hormone adjustment, as well.

A young girl raised on a typical high-fat Western diet has much higher estrogen levels and begins her menstrual cycle at a much younger age than one eating a RAVE Diet. In just 140 years, the average age of puberty in US girls has dropped from 17 to 12 – and menopause starts four years later. In other words, women on high-fat diets have added nine years of menstrual cycles to their lives. How do we know diet causes this? Because women throughout the world, including those in the US, raised on RAVE Diets reach puberty at the normal age of 16 or 17.

When women experience tenderness in their breasts each month, it's because estrogen is stimulating breast cells to divide and that's when a mutation, or cancer cell, is most likely to appear. If you have more menstrual cycles and more stimulation from higher levels of estrogen, there's a much greater chance you'll develop not only breast cancer, but also other hormone-related cancers.

Milk is full of *bovine estrogen* from cows, so it's little wonder that dairy products have been strongly linked to breast and prostate cancer. Body fat also stimulates the production of estrogen, so the more body fat you have, the higher

---

[30] Cancer, January 2002;94:272-281; Cancer, March 2002; 94:1867-75.

your estrogen levels will be. This is the reason overweight women have higher cancer risks.

Pesticides and other chemical toxins also raise estrogen levels because these chemicals mimic sex hormones once they are inside the body. Since 95 percent of the pesticides Americans consume are in meat and dairy products – not plant foods – you're getting a double-boost to your hormone levels when you eat animal foods.

Breast cancer thrives in an estrogen-rich environment and estrogen levels for American women are up to twice as high as women around the world eating low-fat, plant-based diets. The problems American women experience with menopause is due to the *dramatic drop in estrogen levels*. If you get rid of this sharp drop, you get rid of the problems. By changing to the RAVE Diet before you reach menopause, the drop in estrogen levels will be small and smooth – and you will eliminate the problems. The Japanese, for example, don't even have a word for "hot flash" simply because Japanese women eating traditional, plant-based diets do not experience hot flashes – or other problems associated with menopause.

Eating a high-fiber diet is important because fiber removes excessive sex hormones from the body and lowers estrogen levels, greatly reducing your risk of cancer. If these hormones are not carried out by fiber, they are recycled back into the blood, which drives up hormone levels even further.

Men who eat high-fat diets also reach puberty earlier and have abnormally high levels of male sex hormones. Eating animal foods stimulates the production of testosterone. Lowering those levels will prevent prostate cancer and slow the growth of any cancer that has already developed.[31] This knowledge has led to the development of testosterone-lowering drugs for the treatment of prostate cancer, but there's a simpler, cheaper and more powerful way to lower testosterone levels: simply change to a low-fat, high-fiber diet.[32]

Prostate cancer is more strongly related to the consumption of nonfat dairy products than to any other food.[33] In one study, it was shown that high

---

[31] DePrimo SE. Prevention of prostate cancer. Hematol Oncol Clin North Am. 2001 Jun;15(3):445-57; Brawley OW. Prostate cancer prevention trials in the USA. Eur J Cancer. 2000 Jun;36(10):1312-5.

[32] Howie BJ. Dietary and hormonal interrelationships among vegetarian Seventh-Day Adventists and nonvegetarian men. Am J Clin Nutr. 1985 Jul;42(1):127-34; Key TJ. Testosterone, sex hormone-binding globulin, calculated free testosterone, and oestradiol in male vegans and omnivores. Br J Nutr. 1990 Jul;64(1):111-9; Habito RC. Postprandial changes in sex hormones after meals of different composition. Metabolism. 2001 May;50(5):505-11; Belanger A. Influence of diet on plasma steroids and sex hormone-binding globulin levels in adult men. J Steroid Biochem. 1989 Jun;32(6):829-33.

[33] Grant WB. An ecologic study of dietary links to prostate cancer. Altern Med Rev. 1999 Jun;4(3):162-9

consumption of dairy products was associated with a 50 percent increase in the risk of prostate cancer.[34] One possible reason for this involves vitamin D, which is known to protect against cancer. Consuming high levels of calcium, as found in dairy foods, lowers the levels of vitamin D and in doing so, lowers its protective qualities.

Prostate cancer does not occur with men throughout the world who are eating low-fat diets, because they have normal levels of testosterone. While many studies have linked high testosterone levels to prostate cancer, the most revealing fact is that prostate cancer simply does not occur in eunuchs, men castrated at an early age. Incidentally, you'll never see a bald eunuch because hair loss is also related to testosterone levels. Although a tendency toward hair loss is genetic, you can significantly delay its onset and slow or arrest its spread by getting your testosterone level back to normal with a change to the RAVE Diet. In some cases, a change in diet has actually resulted in the re-growth of hair.

Prostate reduction is also linked to a low-fat, plant-based diet and prostate cancer is rare in populations that eat such a diet. Most prostate cancers have decades of slow growth before a tumor develops. This is the time when a change in diet can be most effective in strengthening your immune system and killing those cancer cells. And getting your testosterone level back to normal will not affect your manliness – only your chances of getting cancer – and perhaps going bald before your time.

Eating any farm animal today adds to your hormone overdose because large corporate farms use hormones to increase animal growth and output – and these hormones are passed on to us when we eat these animals or their products. Since 1995, Europe has banned the use of hormones in farm animals because of the links to human cancers. Europe has also banned American beef from its shores because of our continued use of hormones on livestock.

The modern cow produces 25 times more milk than a cow did just 50 years ago. A good part of that increased production is due to drugs, antibiotics – and artificial hormones. In fact, milk turns out to be a hormonal delivery system as it contains over 50 different hormones. Numerous studies have shown links between the hormones in dairy products and the development of hormone-related cancers. In populations eating low-fat RAVE diets, breast, colon, prostate and other cancers are rare or non-existent.

Another mechanism linking dairy with hormonal cancers is the powerful growth-stimulating hormone, known as insulin-like growth factor-1 (IGF-1), which has been strongly linked to the development of cancer of the breast, prostate, lung, and colon because it stimulates cell proliferation and inhibits cell

---

[34] Chan JM. Dairy products, calcium, phosphorous, vitamin D, and risk of prostate cancer (Sweden) Cancer Causes Control. 1998 Dec;9(6):559-66.

death – two activities you don't want when cancer cells are involved.[35] This hormone is increased in the body by the consumption of protein, and especially animal protein. Dairy products stimulate the production of IGF-1 more than any other food.[36]

Years ago, the link between fat and cancer was observed by the Surgeon General, who said that in comparing populations, "...death rates for cancers of the breast, colon, and prostate are directly proportional to estimated dietary fat intakes."[37]

There are many "experts" who say a low-fat diet won't make a dent against cancer. Of course, their version of low fat is a 30 percent fat diet (which is high fat!). A 30 percent fat diet will not only *not* make a dent, it will *cause* breast cancer. You will not prevent the incidence of breast, or our other common cancers, until you cut dietary fat intake down to ten percent of total calories – the same dietary fat level that reverses heart disease.

Conventional Cancer Treatments

"Many medicines few cures." – Benjamin Franklin, Poor Richard's Almanac

"Most cancer patients in this country die of chemotherapy. Chemotherapy does not eliminate breast, colon, or lung cancers. This fact has been documented for over a decade, yet doctors still use chemotherapy for these tumors."
Allen Levin, M.D., UCSF, The Healing of Cancer

"There are three kinds of lies in the world: lies, damn lies, and statistics."
Benjamin Disraeli

The medical profession looks quizzically on "spontaneous" cancer remissions, cancers that have disappeared for no apparent reason. But upon close inspection, it's been found that almost 90 percent of these "spontaneous" remissions occurred after people made big changes to their diets,[38] changes which strengthened their immune systems.

---

[35] Yu H. Role of the insulin-like growth factor family in cancer development and progression. J Natl Cancer Inst. 2000 Sep 20;92(18):1472-89.

[36] Holmes MD. Dietary Correlates of Plasma Insulin-like Growth Factor I and Insulin-like Growth Factor Binding Protein 3 Concentrations. Cancer Epidemiol Biomarkers Prev 2002 Sep;11(9):852-61.

[37] U.S. Department of Health and Human Services. Surgeon General's Report on Nutrition and Health. DHHS Publ No. 88-50210, 1988.

[38] Lifestyle Changes and the 'Spontaneous' Regression of Cancer..., Foster, H, Inter. Jnl Biosocial Research, 10(1), 1988, pp. 17-33, as quoted in Reclaiming Our Health, John Robbins, p. 283.

Conventional treatments do not cure cancer.[39] In fact, they severely damage your only hope of curing the cancer – the immune system. Following conventional treatments, cancer remains in the body. When the doctors say they got all of it, they are not telling you the whole story because there can be over a *million* cancer cells in your body they cannot detect, just waiting for an opportunity to regroup and multiply in order to resume their lethal march. The fact they did not get it all is one reason for such a high rate of cancer recurrence. Only the immune system is smart enough to selectively recognize cancer cells and completely cure cancer. After conventional treatments, however, the immune system is so damaged it is not surprising that cancers re-emerge so frequently.

Despite what you've read in the news, the success rate for breast cancer, for example, *has not changed over the last 80 years*. Women with breast cancer do not live longer, after they have been diagnosed, than they did in the 1920s – and over 90 percent of the women diagnosed with breast cancer will die of breast cancer. Despite ever-aggressive treatments and early detection, the expected increase in life expectancy with conventional treatments is close to zero. In fact, when conventional treatments are used, life extension is a matter of only months, not years, compared to those who did not receive treatment.[40]

The cancer success rates you hear about in the news are due primarily to statistical manipulation as a result of increases in "five-year survival" rates. This increase, however, is due solely to early detection – which simply means that the clock measuring "five year survival" starts running sooner, *not that patients live any longer*. In other words, the improvement in survival rates is merely a statistical deception. The patient "lives longer" within the five-year clock, simply because the clock starts sooner due to early detection.

The cancer industry becomes giddy as the media promotes early detection because the earlier the detection, the greater the five-year survival rates will be, which makes the cancer industry look as if it is actually helping people. But, in fact, all the cancer industry has done is made people's lives miserable by putting them through surgery, chemotherapy, radiation and other invasive treatments – and created a living hell for patients through nausea, vomiting, infections and damage to their internal organs – while pocketing billions of dollars. And after all this "treatment," they have not extended the lives of their patients one iota. In those few "successful" cases, most cancer patients die of a later recurrence of cancer or a disease brought on by the chemotherapy or radiation treatments themselves. In fact, if you add in all the people who have died of another disease

---

[39] For an in-depth analysis of this, see the book Healing Cancer From Inside Out by Mike Anderson.

[40] The following studies show that untreated patients lived as long, if not longer then treated patients: JAMA, 1992, 257, p. 2191; Lancet, 1991, August, p. 901; NEJM, 1986, May 8, p. 1226; NEJM, 1984, March, p. 737; Cancer, 1981, 47, p. 27; JAMA, 1979;241:489-494 ; A Report on Cancer, 1969, Hardin Jones.

because of the side effects of chemotherapy and radiation (e.g., died of pneumonia due to a weakened immune system), conventional treatments have done far more harm than good.

In plain English, cancer victims would have lived the same number of years without conventional treatments. The sad fact is that people are not living longer as a result of conventional treatments, they are just being given a longer death sentence. The next time you hear about improvements in cancer treatments, ask for improvements in life expectancy rates, not five-year survival rates. You could survive conventional treatments for five years and die in the sixth year and the cancer industry would consider their treatments a success – and record it as such. Don't fall for this statistical lie.

The origins of chemotherapy are found in chemical warfare agents, such as mustard gas, and chemotherapy is just as toxic to the patient as it is to the enemy soldier it was intended for. All the cancer industry did was turn chemo-warfare into chemo-therapy and coin the term "war on cancer."

Regardless of the name (Tamoxifen, Herceptin, etc.), all chemotherapeutic treatments do much more harm than good for the body and they have not proven to be successful in either curing cancer or extending lives.

Back in 1985, an article in the *Scientific American* showed that chemotherapy was able to "save" the lives of, at most, just three percent of cancer patients.[41]

In 1990, a renowned biostatistics expert reviewed chemotherapy-treated cancer patients and concluded that chemo can help only about three percent of patients with epithelial cancers, such as breast, prostate, colon and lung cancers.[42]

In 2006, a comprehensive review of chemotherapy treatments in the U.S. and Australia from 1990 to 2004 on 22 of our most common cancers, showed that once again, chemotherapy contributed to survival rates in only three percent of patients![43] And these were only five-year survival rates!

The medical profession generally considers any drug with less than 30 percent effectiveness no better than a placebo. So how, you might ask, can the medical profession get away with using chemotherapy when the results are downright pathetic and far less than what you would expect using a placebo?

The answer, once again, is statistics.

If a doctor were to say that by giving you toxic chemotherapy treatments, your survival rate would increase from three to six percent, I think you would reply, "I'd rather visit a witch doctor!" However, the presentation doesn't follow that path. Instead, oncologists turn the statistic around. If a treatment causes survival

---

[41] The Treatment of Diseases and the War Against Cancer, John Cairns, Scientific American, 253(5), Nov. 1985.

[42] Abel Urich, Chemotherapy of Advanced Epithelial Cancer: A Critical Survey, Hippokrates Verlag Stuttgart, 1990.

[43] The contribution of cytotoxic chemotherapy to 5-year survival in adult malignancies, Morgan G, Ward R, Barton M., Clin Oncol (R Coll Radiol). 2004;16(8):549-60.

rates to increase from three percent to six percent, well, that represents a 50 percent increase in survival rates! That is exactly the sales pitch the medical profession uses to convince people to follow chemo treatments. You are told that this wonderful new chemotherapy drug can actually increase your chances of survival by a whopping 50 percent, not the measly two or six percent! Now what patient wouldn't risk trying that drug with those percentages? Unfortunately, the foundation of the entire cancer industry rests on these statistical deceptions and they keep hitting the news every week.

Much the same can be said for radiation treatments, which are also extremely toxic to the body. Does it not seem strange to you that we are trying to cure cancers with a treatment that has been proven to cause cancers?

Instead of allowing the body to take care of cancer cells naturally by strengthening the immune system, we assault the body with invasive and destructive agents of war. Our current arsenal of cancer treatments is the modern equivalent of bloodletting because in these cases, the "cure" is all too often worse than the disease. The truly remarkable thing is how the body can survive these treatments at all. Even the medical establishment has acknowledged the failure of cancer treatments. In the February 9, 1994 issue of the *Journal of the American Medical Association*, the "War on Cancer" was declared a failure. "In all age groups, cancer incidence is increasing…few new effective treatments have been devised for the most common cancers."

What would I do if I had cancer? I would investigate every natural cure for cancer that strengthens the immune system and cleanses the body of toxins. I would never subject myself to conventional treatments that destroy the only hope of curing cancer – the immune system. To be sure, there are people running cancer-cure scams, but there are also legitimate institutions, which take patients who have been given death warrants by conventional medicine – and these institutions have brought patients back to robust health and long lives.

Why doesn't mainstream medicine embrace these treatments, despite their successes? Simply because natural treatments are not attractive candidates for investment, due to the fact they are *not patentable* and therefore *not profitable.* Sadly, when natural treatments score solid cancer successes and have a strong track record, they are dismissed as dubious quackery. When an extremely toxic but potentially profitable drug can show only marginal rates of success, however, it will easily enter the realm of "acceptable treatments."

If you are skeptical that profitability is the prime decision-making criteria for mainstream cancer treatments, please pick up a copy of *Healing Cancer From Inside Out* by this author, available as both a book and film.

Also, check our web site for a current list of institutions that treat cancers naturally. (www.RAVEDiet.com) The web site also contains many personal stories of people completely curing life-threatening cancers, as well as other diseases, by adopting a RAVE-like diet and lifestyle.

Take the case of Anthony Sattilaro, M.D., who contracted prostate cancer and it rapidly spread throughout his body. He was just 46 years old when his oncologist told him the cancer had gone too far, there was nothing he could do, and Dr. Sattilaro should prepare to die.

A few days after this pronouncement, Dr. Sattilaro happened across two young men looking for a ride and he decided to give them one. In their discussion, Dr. Sattilaro mentioned the death sentence he was facing. The two men happened to be attending a macrobiotic cooking school and told him that if he changed his diet, the cancer would go away.

You can imagine how an M.D. would feel about getting cancer advice from two young kids! The boys asked for his address and later sent him more information. The information could not satisfy his scientific standards, but he was driven by a combination of curiosity and desperation. After all, conventional medicine had given up on him. What did he have to lose?

He went to a meeting and decided then that he would adopt the diet. The tastes were different than what he had been used to, but he decided to stick with the diet because of one significant thing, which started happening very soon after he switched his eating habits: *The terrible pain he was suffering started to diminish!* He found he needed less pain medication and *in just three weeks* his cancer pain was completely gone. His energy returned and he was able to work again. He continued on what was essentially an Asian peasant's diet with large amounts of brown rice and vegetables, while strictly avoiding all dairy, meat and refined foods.

A year later, he went to his doctor and asked to be re-tested for cancer. When the results came back, his doctors were shocked. The cancer was gone. It was no longer in his bones, his spine, his skull nor anywhere else in his body.

For the next ten years, Dr. Sattilaro led a life that was cancer free. He got so involved in diet that he wrote a book about his experience, entitled *Recalled by Life*. Then something unfortunate happened. After ten years of a cancer-free existence, he decided to re-introduce fish and chicken into his diet. Shortly thereafter, the cancer returned, along with the pain. Despite ten years of being declared free of cancer following his change in diet, his medical mind was still not totally convinced the diet had made the difference. As a result, he continued eating chicken and fish, was forced to resume taking his narcotic painkillers – and soon the cancer killed him.

A woman contracted breast cancer and cured it by using natural treatments and adopting a RAVE-like diet.[44] Years after her cancer was gone – thinking she was somehow now immune from cancer – she decided to return to her previous diet – of chicken and fish. Just like Dr. Sattilaro, soon after she changed back to her old diet, breast cancer showed up for the second time. Unlike Dr. Sattilaro, however, she switched back to a RAVE-like diet and underwent natural treatments for a

---

[44] Triumph Over Cancer, Agi Lidle.

second time. Fortunately, her breast cancer vanished once again. She had learned her lesson about the power of diet for the last time.

These are just two stories, but there are thousands more, which demonstrate just how *powerful* a big change in diet and lifestyle can be.

Within the next few years, cancer is expected to eclipse heart disease as the number one cause of death in America. It is already the number one fear, and rightly so because we have no effective treatment for cancer and no medical cure.

The average American has six bouts with serious cancers during their lifetimes. Those with healthy immune systems won't even know about the battle their bodies are waging with cancer. Those with weakened immune systems will find out about their battle in the hospital.

Each and every immune cell is made from the food you eat. A deficient diet means a deficient immune system. Nurture your immune system with the RAVE Diet & Lifestyle and it will protect you against not only our common cancers, but our other major diseases, as well.

Other Diet-Related Diseases

There are many other diseases that can be cured with simple changes in diet. One lady recently adopted the RAVE Diet and her arthritis was completely gone after just three months. And so were the drugs she had been taking for decades. Did her doctor ever mention a change in diet to her? Of course not. He was totally baffled. He wasn't even aware diet could do this – until *she* told him.

The problem with modern medicine is that our authorities are completely unaware of the power of diet. As mentioned previously, studies will change the fat content of diets from 40 percent to 30 percent with no effect. But small changes like this will not cure anything. And based on such worthless studies, medical practitioners will tell you diet plays no role in diseases.

Unfortunately, these studies have not gone far enough and the medical establishment simply doesn't get it. Women eating RAVE Diets do not get breast cancer. Men eating RAVE Diets do not get prostate cancer. Nor do they get any of the other common eating-related cancers or other diseases, such as heart disease. They don't become overweight, and they don't get diabetes, arthritis or hundreds of other diseases now plaguing Americans. In fact, our eating habits have become so bad that children are now being diagnosed with *adult* diabetes.

"The disease as we know it really has no cure right now." – Marie T. Allen, Director of the Navajo Nation, Special Diabetes Project

The American Diabetes Association will also tell you there is no cure for adult-onset diabetes, but that simply means there is no drug that will "cure" the disease. They are simply wrong because adult-onset diabetes is easily cured – and quickly – cured with a change of diet and lifestyle.

Dr. Joel Fuhrman reports that over 90 percent of his patients who were on insulin at the time of their first visit, were taken *completely off their medications within the first month*![45] Numerous clinics have stated that under their care they can get diabetics completely off insulin in just a week.[46] In fact, Dr. Fuhrman has called insulin the worst thing to ever happen to diabetics because it keeps them on an eating habit that caused the disease in the first place.

Many think that simply taking drugs, such as insulin, will enable them to tolerate the disease while making no changes in their diet, but long term use of any drug will eventually take its toll on the body. And recent studies have shown that diabetes treatment actually does more harm than good![47]

Virtually all cases of adult-onset diabetes can be completely reversed with diet – and most within a matter of a few months or sooner. Even the few who cannot get off their medications can benefit from the RAVE Diet because their medications will be drastically reduced. Even Type I diabetics can have their medications reduced by a third by following the RAVE Diet.[48]

Check our web site (www.RaveDiet.com) because it has many personal stories of people curing life-threatening diseases by adopting a RAVE Diet & Lifestyle. Diseases ranging from rheumatoid arthritis to lupus to cancers have all been reversed following RAVE diets.

Due to the long time span involved in degenerative diseases, researchers are still trying to unravel the causes of such diseases, but diet is at the heart of all of them. Take a simple condition such as acne, which affects up to 95 percent of all American teenagers. Currently, the medical profession confidently states that diet plays no role in acne. However, there are many studies of teenagers *in other countries* who eat native diets of whole plant foods where acne is simply unknown. *Not a single teenager gets acne.*[49] Western medicine needs to cast its net wider and look at people eating non-Western diets before they conclude that diet plays no role in diseases.

---

[45] Eat To Live, Joel Fuhrman, M.D., p. 6.

[46] Testimonies provided in the films *Eating* and *Healing Cancer From Inside Out* by Mike Anderson.

[47] Duckworth W, et al. Glucose Control and Vascular Complications in Veterans with Type 2 Diabetes. N Engl J Med. 2008 Dec 17. (Epub date); Action to Control Cardiovascular Risk in Diabetes Study Group, Gerstein HC, et al. Effects of intensive glucose lowering in type 2 diabetes. N Engl J Med. 2008 Jun 12;358(24):2545-59.

[48] John A. McDougall, M.D., www.drmcdougall.com/science/diabetes.html.

[49] Acne vulgaris: a disease of Western civilization, Cordain L., Arch Dermatol. 2002 Dec;138(12):1584-90; Acne diet reconsidered, Rosenberg EW, Arch Dermatol. 1981 Apr;117(4):193-5; Western Culture May Be Culprit Behind Acne, Reuters Health, 12/20/02; Diet may trigger acne after all, Los Angeles Times, 1/6/03.

Weight Loss Using Old-Fashioned Foods

The fundamental trick to successful weight loss is to figure out a way to eat fewer calories, while feeling full and satisfied.

The problem with modern diets is that we consume far too many calories before we feel full. We then try to reduce calories by reducing portion sizes, which makes us feel deprived, if not downright depraved. This is precisely why modern diets fail in the long run. Yes, you can lose weight by reducing portion sizes, but you don't feel quite human doing it day-in and day-out, year after year. There is something intrinsically wrong with this approach and the reason modern diets are such failures. Among many other things, it sets up the yo-yo cycle of dietary restriction, then failure and binge eating, so you end up gaining more weight than if you had never started dieting in the first place.

The RAVE Diet approaches diet in a different manner. In the first place, the root of the word "diet" means lifestyle and, since your body is the most obvious and visible feature of your life, if you want to change your body, you're going to have to change your life – and change it for good. By following all aspects of the RAVE Diet, your life will be transformed.

The RAVE Diet is also linear in that most people will start out eating what I call "transition" or substitution foods (see *Transition Foods*) until they fully adopt the RAVE Diet. This allows a smooth transition into the full-blown RAVE Diet and hopefully avoids the yo-yo syndrome. This is not a crash diet to lose lots of weight in three weeks (although it can be, depending on you), but a gradual approach to changing your eating and living habits so you can not only live with the foods you eat, but live with yourself. The rate of weight loss really depends on how much you have to lose. If you are interested in losing weight fast, see *Accelerating Weight Loss*. (If you are trying to reverse a disease, however, you should be on the full RAVE Diet, without any transition foods.)

Remember the hare and tortoise story in the beginning? The tortoise always wins when it comes to losing weight. The RAVE Diet will accommodate lapses in eating because it requires that you change your *attitude* about eating. Once your attitude has changed, you may fall off the horse occasionally, but you'll have the knowledge and confidence to know you'll get back on it and ride again.

The RAVE Diet is really a throwback to the old-fashioned diets our ancestors ate. Before the early 1800's, modern refined foods were not readily available, yet today, refined foods occupy over 50 percent of our calories. Eating animal foods, including dairy products, was a very occasional event due to a lack of availability (no refrigeration and high cost). Today, animal foods constitute a whopping 40 percent of our total calories. Taken together, *over 90 percent of the calories we consume today are from foods that were either non-existent back then or were eaten only on special occasions.*

Today, only seven percent of our calories come from natural, whole plant foods, yet these were the foods where the bulk of our ancestors calories came from, in the form of whole grain breads, potatoes, brown rice, corn, oats, rye, barley meals, beans and other vegetables, fruits and whole grains.

When the eating habits of numerous populations are compared, the results are strikingly consistent: As the consumption of natural plant foods declined, there was a corresponding rise in diet-related diseases, including weight gain.[50] When almost all their calories came from natural, whole plant foods, there was almost never a problem with weight, nor diet-related diseases. The one exception was the wealthy, which could afford to eat the way Americans eat today.

In other words, the RAVE Diet calls upon you to look back at the foods your ancestors ate – and make their past habits your future habits. Unrefined, old-fashioned foods are better because whole foods fill you up on fewer calories, whereas modern processed foods require that you eat excessive calories before you feel full – the reason we're gaining weight.[51]

Of course, you could run 10 miles a day and you would lose weight no matter what kind of diet you were eating. But would you be healthy? You might *look* healthy, but despite your weight loss, you might not be healthy on the inside. We all know the famous cases of long-distance runners who dropped dead of heart attacks. That's because their coronary arteries were clogged due to their diets. In the case of Jim Fixx, for example, his coronary arteries were plugged solid with atherosclerosis. One was 99 percent blocked, another 80 percent, and a third 70 percent. Losing weight isn't a problem. Losing weight and staying healthy is.

This old-fashioned RAVE Diet will fill you up without restricting portions, reduce your caloric intake gradually, never leave you hungry and always leave you healthy. The only things you'll be deprived of on this diet are the major diseases that are wreaking havoc on American health today.

Why Doesn't The Government Promote This Diet?

There is an overwhelming amount of scientific and other data that tells us the RAVE Diet is the healthiest diet on the planet. With Americans getting sicker each day from the foods we eat, you might be asking, "If this diet is so great, why doesn't the government promote it?"

Good question. First of all, the government "does" promote it, but in a very miniscule way. If you compare what the government spends promoting whole plant foods versus what it spends promoting animal and refined foods, I doubt it would amount to a tenth of one percent. Compared to the billions of dollars spent

---

[50] Eat To Live, Joel Fuhrman, M.D., p. 51.
[51] Trends in Intake of Energy and Macronutrients --- United States, 1971—2000, Centers For Disease Control, February 6, 2004 / 53(04);80-82.

subsidizing the meat, dairy, egg and sugar industries, for example, fruits and vegetables destined for human consumption receive zero subsidies. (Even feed crops destined for *farm animal* consumption receive subsidies, but those destined for human consumption do not. This, of course, is the result of meat and dairy industry lobbying.)

When the US changed to an animal-based diet early in the 1900s, everyone thought animal foods (meat, egg and dairy products) were nutritionally beneficial. In fact, the government got behind meat and dairy farmers and started promoting these foods to help farmers out which were, at the time, very small businesses. One of the key missions of the U.S. Dept. of Agriculture is, in fact, to promote meat and dairy products and it continues to do so to this day. The "Got Milk?" and "Beef, it's what's for dinner," and "Pork, the other white meat," as well as a myriad of other advertising campaigns, are all government-sponsored programs. The federally-funded school breakfast and lunch programs are simply subsidized dumping grounds for unhealthy food designed to put money into corporate pockets regardless of what it is doing to the health of the school children forced to eat that garbage.

Today, small farmers have been displaced by huge agri-businesses that receive almost all agricultural subsidies – and reap almost all the profits. And to ensure that the tradition of political support and rich subsidies continues uninterrupted, agri-businesses funnel millions of dollars into the pockets of politicians every election.

With the democratization of animal foods (and refrigerators), everyone thought Americans had the best darn diet on the planet because rich foods were affordable and everyone could eat animal products on a regular basis. At mid-point in the century, however, something started to happen to Americans – they were suddenly dying of heart attacks and cancer was starting to spread like wildfire.

Since we had the best diet on the planet, no one suspected that eating animal foods had anything to do with these two health epidemics. Medical researchers searched high and low for an explanation and came up empty-handed – until a few researchers started looking into our change to an animal-based diet.

Once the investigation into diet showed promise, massive efforts were employed in an attempt to find out what it was about our diet that caused disease. Over 50 years later, we are literally buried in scientific papers linking animal foods to the leading causes of death and disability in this country.

"Okay," you might be saying. "But with all this evidence, why doesn't the government do something?" In a phrase: money and politics. The meat and dairy industries are a huge part of the economy. They contribute massive amounts of campaign finance money in very successful efforts to purchase politicians. The politicians think this is good because it not only allows them to get re-elected, but also because these food industries employ people, which helps keep our economy going. So our politicians continue to subsidize these industries that would, in fact, go bankrupt without these subsidies. Ironically, the meat, egg and dairy industries are the same people who tout freedom of the marketplace and want *no* government interference in their businesses, except when it comes to receiving subsidies or promoting their products. In that case, government corruption of the marketplace is quite all right.

Along with our change in diet, came a change in taste, which has continued through the generations. Americans now crave animal foods. When meat prices go up, as they did during the Nixon administration, there is a howl of protest from consumers, who demanded that politicians do something.

The end result is a joining of several forces that effectively block any attempt to change things. Consumers love their meat and politicians love the money they get from agri-businesses. The government gives only lip service to healthy foods because, quite frankly, there is no profit – or political payoff – in such foods. In addition, the pharmaceutical and medical industries would not be the giants they are today were it not for our diet. In other words, these industries have no incentive to change things, either – and both contribute heavily to our politicians.

The last time we saw a report on Nutrition and Health by the Surgeon General was back in 1988. It was supposed to be updated every two years, but the report's damnation of dietary fat created so much furor with food lobbies that our politicians effectively censored any further reports from that office.

Despite the report's indictment of animal food, people who worked on the report were told, in no uncertain terms, that the report's recommendations could not say, "eat less meat."[52] So instead of saying, "eat less meat," agencies found a way to water down their recommendations by saying, "eat less saturated fat." This was acceptable to the meat lobby because it means far less to the consumer than saying, "eat less meat." This language compromise has led to a great deal of confusion in the public mind. Health agencies would like to say, "eat less meat," because that has meaning to consumers, but their hands are tied by food industry influence. This is the primary reason you see health authorities today saying "eat less saturated fat" – because it is politically correct and does not threaten their own sources of income from food industries.

The influence of food industries spreads much further than Washington. In fact, food industries deliberately contribute money to health organizations in order to water down their nutritional recommendations. It's now become a part of their marketing strategy, just like advertising. The health organizations to which food industries contribute include the likes of the American Cancer Society, the American Heart Association and the American Dietetic Association,[53] as well as individual health authorities who have any influence over the public. In addition, food industries contribute millions of dollars every year to universities that do studies for them that are designed to sell their products.

---

[52] Food Politics, Marion Nestle, p. 3.
[53] Food Politics, Marion Nestle, p. 113.

Food industries spend a tremendous amount of money on advertising not just in television and print media, but in medical and nutritional journals. As a result, their editorial influence is pervasive in terms of what gets said and printed in the media. These industries also employ an army of professional writers who are skilled at writing letters to the editor or reviews of books on Amazon.com. It's more than likely the next time you see a letter to an editor touting the benefits of one animal food or another, or criticizing plant-based diets, that letter was written by a hired gun from a food lobby.

Some public figures will rail against any government interference when it comes to food choices and shout there must be "freedom of choice" when it comes to food. In fact, however, we have no freedom of choice because politicians in Washington have already decided what Americans are going to eat. By subsidizing the animal and refined food industries, the heavy hand of the government has already interfered in the marketplace and made hamburger – one of the most expensive and resource-intensive foods on the planet – cheaper than raspberries. Until such subsidies are gone and the government gets out of food price-fixing, the "freedom of choice" argument is empty. We have no free market or freedom of choice when it comes to food.

The only way we are going to make Americans eat healthy food is by letting the free market determine the price of food. That means taking away all subsidies received by food industries by voting for campaign finance reform. A free market would make unhealthy foods so expensive, only the wealthy could afford to eat them – and die from them – on a regular basis. If those subsidies could be "willed away" overnight, our eating habits would be back in the 18th century and our diets would resemble the old-fashioned diets of our ancestors, who did not suffer from the diet-related diseases that are ravaging us today. Degenerative diseases would vanish from the landscape, just as they did when the Nazis removed animal foods from the countries it occupied.

Of course, you don't have to wait for the government to do this. You can do this yourself by simply following the RAVE Diet.

I was recently at an American Heart Association fund-raiser. I really wasn't surprised when I found out the main course was veal (I opted for their meat-less entrée). Serving veal or prime rib or some other form of meat is typical of "health" organizations. Why do they serve such unhealthy fare? Because they are trying to raise money – and unwittingly – bring more heart patients into the hospital because the more heart patients in hospitals, the more money they will raise for research into treating a disease that could be completely cured by simple changes in diet. In fact, we do not need any further research into heart disease. We already have a cure for heart disease. It is diet.

Baseline Measurements: Countering Skepticism

"You can fool some of the people all of the time, and all of the people some of the time, but you cannot fool all of the people all of the time." – Abraham Lincoln

It's difficult to convince many people that diet can be so powerful. Most eating diseases are like nutritional time-bombs which take decades to develop, so people may feel healthy now, but they no doubt have heart disease, cancer and other diseases slowly growing in their bodies.

I remember talking to a woman who was very skeptical of the RAVE Diet. She said, "Look at me! I'm healthy and I eat whatever I want!" She, like so many other people, considered herself as healthy as her peers. Unfortunately, being as healthy as one's peers in American is not being healthy at all. She was grossly overweight (she called it a few extra pounds) and I could tell by just looking at her – and generally knowing what she ate – that she suffered from at least heart disease and no doubt other diseases were at work inside her body. A few years after our brief conversation, I learned through a mutual friend that she had a heart attack. Don't let *your* skepticism keep you from this diet just because you're as healthy as your peers. Our norms for what is healthy have steadily deteriorated over the years and these norms are killing people.

There are many claims being made by various diet plans, which would make anyone skeptical. If you are a "normally healthy" – and skeptical – person and want to try the RAVE Diet, what I would suggest is that you test your own skepticism by getting a few tests done *before* you start the diet, then re-test in six months (or earlier). That will be a measure of just how healthy your skepticism really was.

A friend of mine was on the Atkins diet for many years and was very skeptical of the RAVE Diet. He did lose some weight on Atkins, but it crept back over the years until he was back where he started. He continued with Atkins until his doctors discovered his coronary arteries were blocked. They put a stent in, which served as his wake-up call, so he finally started the RAVE Diet. He lost 80 pounds and he's never felt better. His test results are now the best they have ever been in his life and his total cholesterol is at 116. His cardiologists are amazed and somewhat baffled. He now thinks they are incompetent. I would not go that far. They are very skilled at manipulating drugs, performing surgeries and providing temporary fixes for a broken heart. But the typical cardiologist does not have a clue how to actually *cure* heart disease. In fact, most of them are on Lipitor! Sadly, by the time you finish this book, you'll know more about curing heart disease than your doctor does.

The RAVE Diet heals internally and aside from weight loss (if you're overweight), you won't be able to "see" how your body is healing without these tests. Once your test results come back, you'll not only be amazed, but your doctor will, too. Another friend of mine adopted the RAVE Diet and her cholesterol dropped 60 points in just three weeks. All her doctor could say was "I don't know what you're doing, but keep doing it." The truly sad part is that the doctor should have given her this dietary advice, not me.

The following should be goals to make sure you are heart-attack proof. And these are goals that should be met without any medication.

Total Cholesterol:	below 150
LDL:	below 90
Triglycerides:	below 150
Homocystein:	below 10
Blood Pressure:	110/70 – 125/80
Weight:	Ideal/Good

Don't worry about your total cholesterol getting too low. Despite what you may have heard, this has never happened to any human being. The typical rural Chinese peasant has total cholesterol levels around 80 – 90 and they would consider a total cholesterol level of 150 to be very high. Of course, with the introduction of American food in Chinese cities, Chinese cholesterol levels are skyrocketing, along with their diet-related diseases.

It should be mentioned that a recent study made headlines by claiming that low cholesterol is somehow linked to (and caused) cancer.[54] Nothing could be further from the truth! In fact, some cancers *cause* low cholesterol levels because they impair the liver's ability to produce cholesterol. The people in the study who had very low cholesterol levels had undiagnosed cancers. Their low cholesterol levels were the result of their cancer, not the other way around.

Despite the efficacy of these tests, they are still only markers, i.e., they do not measure the blood flow to the heart, i.e., how plugged up your arteries may be. For those truly concerned about their heart condition, you can get any number of tests that measure blood flow to the heart, e.g., a Thallium stress test or MUGA scan. Your doctor can tell you which test is the best for you.

Note: In the beginning, your HDL ("good cholesterol") will go up because you are getting rid of excess cholesterol and clearing your arteries. HDL is a measure of the cholesterol leaving your body. Over time, however, the HDL will go *down* because there will simply be less cholesterol to get rid of, since you are not consuming it, nor high levels of saturated fat. Ideally, the ratio of total cholesterol to HDL should be less than 3. (Divide your total cholesterol by your HDL, e.g.,

---

[54] Yang X, WingYee S,Ko GT. Independent associations between low-density lipoprotein cholesterol and cancer among patients with type 2 diabetes mellitus. CMAJ 2008;179(5):427-437.

150 total cholesterol / 50 HDL = 3.)[55] The point is, you should really be more concerned about your LDL ("bad cholesterol"), not HDL. This is the reason HDL is not listed, above, as a measurable goal.

Weight Measurements

Your current weight is the single best indicator of what your future health is going to be like, so it's important to get it under control. Below are general weight tables for people between 4'10" and 6'3". The ideal weight ranges are best for preventing disease, living at optimal health and adding years to your life. For every pound you are above your ideal weight, your risk of developing diseases rises accordingly.

These are very general ranges for *all* body frames, including men and women. If you want to fine-tune your ideal weight, use a Body Mass Index (BMI) calculator that can take into account frame size. Also, use a BMI calculator to look up your weight if you're outside the height ranges shown here. Healthy weights will also vary depending on your body-fat mass and lean body mass, i.e., if you have a high ratio of lean muscle to fat, you can be above these ranges and still be within your targeted weight range.

The first reaction by many people is that the ideal weight ranges are too "skinny." Quite honestly, this is because we're used to seeing fat people and our perception of what is attractive has changed as the majority of Americans have become overweight. As you lose weight and move close to your ideal weight, your friends will likely be concerned that something is wrong with your health. Actually, it's just the opposite. Something is wrong with *their* health and it revolves around their weight. When I first started doin' the RAVE, I lost 35 pounds in six months and received similar reactions. But while friends were fretting about my "skinny" appearance, they were also full of envy as they peppered me with questions about *how* I lost so much weight – and kept it off.

Ideal

4'10"	91–105	5' 7"	121–140
4'11"	94–109	5' 8"	125–144
5' 0"	97–112	5' 9"	128–149
5' 1"	100–116	5'10"	132–153
5' 2"	104–120	5'11"	136–157
5' 3"	107–124	6' 0"	140–162
5' 4"	110–128	6' 1"	144–166
5' 5"	114–132	6' 2"	148–171
5' 6"	118–136	6' 3"	152–176

[55] Dr. Dean Ornish's Program for Reversing Heart Disease, Dean Ornish, M.D., p. 262.

Good

4'10"	105–119	5' 7"	140–159
4'11"	109–124	5' 8"	144–164
5' 0"	112–128	5' 9"	149–169
5' 1"	116–132	5'10"	153–174
5' 2"	120–136	5'11"	157–179
5' 3"	124–141	6' 0"	162–184
5' 4"	128–145	6' 1"	166–189
5' 5"	132–150	6' 2"	163–194
5' 6"	136–155	6' 3"	176–200

Overweight

4'10"	119–143	5' 7"	159–191
4'11"	124–148	5' 8"	164–197
5' 0"	128–153	5' 9"	169–203
5' 1"	132–158	5'10"	174–209
5' 2"	136–164	5'11"	179–215
5' 3"	141–169	6' 0"	184–221
5' 4"	145–174	6' 1"	189–227
5' 5"	150–180	6' 2"	194–233
5' 6"	155–186	6' 3"	200–240

Obese

4'10"	143+	5' 7"	191+
4'11"	148+	5' 8"	197+
5' 0"	153+	5' 9"	203+
5' 1"	158+	5'10"	209+
5' 2"	164+	5'11"	215+
5' 3"	169+	6' 0"	221+
5' 4"	174+	6' 1"	227+
5' 5"	180+	6' 2"	233+
5' 6"	186+	6' 3"	240+

If your doctor thinks these goals are not realistic, you're seeing the wrong doctor. Go to our web site and see our current list of Healthcare Providers, who can achieve these goals solely through diet and exercise, not drugs.

Practically all adult Americans – and most school children – have heart disease and most adult Americans have cancers slowly growing inside them that can't be detected yet. You can start to reverse these and other diseases by following the

RAVE Diet on your own. If you need assistance with treating a serious disease with diet, again see the list of Healthcare Providers at our web site (www.RaveDiet.com) who regularly heal patients with a wide range of diseases using diet and exercise.

The RAVE Diet & Lifestyle
The Best Health Insurance You Can't Buy

"It turned out to be a lot easier than I had expected. In fact, it felt rather natural. I discovered a new world of foods that were very tasty, diverse, and satisfying. I never felt deprived and, unlike my experiences with other "diets" I had been on, I never felt hungry. Gradually my tastes and orientation to food changed and my desire for the higher-fat foods I had been used to went away." - Raymond Kurzweil, The 10% Solution

21 Days To a New You!

The RAVE Diet is not about restricting food portions, but *changing food choices* and breaking through the vicious eating cycles that are making people sick and overweight. Many people will look at the RAVE Diet and make a snap judgment that it's difficult to follow. It only seems that way. Some of our greatest skeptics decided to try it and found the diet not only easy to follow, but satisfying and delicious.

When we say "21 days to a new you!" we're not talking about losing 21 pounds in 21 days, but *changing your tastes for food in just three weeks*. That's how long it takes most people to make a complete switch in their taste buds. The problem is that we've lost our taste for natural foods because most of the food we eat today is smothered with salt, fat, sweets and chemicals. As a result, our taste buds have become warped as we crave the "highs" of sugar, fat and salt that have become a standard part of the typical American diet. In other words, our taste buds are really driving our diseases.

By following the RAVE Diet, your taste buds will be "re-trained" and the cravings you have for bad foods will be replaced with a desire to eat good food. This is the essence of the RAVE Diet: simply re-training your taste buds to enjoy the foods nature provided for us throughout the history of humanity. Once your taste buds are re-oriented, weight loss and all the other health benefits of this diet will fall into place automatically as your body begins to heal itself.

Many people made a switch from whole milk to skim milk. Do you remember how terrible skim milk tasted when you first tried it? After you got used to it, and you tried whole milk again, remember how awful it tasted? Too heavy, too greasy and too fatty. You will experience similar changes in taste when switching to the RAVE Diet. The highs of sugar, fat, sweets and chemical additives will be replaced by more subtle tastes, along with the aromatic flavors of herbs, spices and sauces. Food will taste so much cleaner – much like the difference between spring water and a syrupy soda.

The RAVE Diet is actually pretty simple in terms of re-training your taste buds because we're already familiar with most of the foods in the diet. The big difference is that we have to eat more of them, then gradually try out unfamiliar foods and discover interesting new tastes.

Your tastes for food will change with this diet and you'll find you prefer the cleaner taste of natural foods. After eating this way, you'll find that high-fat foods will taste heavy and greasy. Many people have told me that when they do eat high-fat foods, their entire system slows down and they feel sluggish.

Stick to the RAVE Diet for 21 days and you'll find you won't want to go back to the heavy, calorie-dense foods you've been eating. In just 21 days, your tastes will change, you'll be on your way to permanent weight loss and you'll be feeling better to boot!

"Progress is very important and exciting – in everything but food." Andy Warhol

Imagine moving to a country where everything is pretty much the same as what we have here – all the modern conveniences, technology, transportation, nice housing, and so forth. But there is one big difference. The way people eat is old-fashioned. They don't have refined foods. They don't allow fiber and cancer-fighting nutrients to be removed from foods. They don't squeeze fruits and vegetables in order to eat concentrated oils from them, while throwing away the rest. And they don't eat the animals they live with. As a result, people live long, healthy, high-quality lives. If you can imagine such a country, it's possible to live there without even moving – by simply adopting the RAVE Diet & Lifestyle.

Today, scientists, pharmaceutical companies, doctors and laymen are all looking for magic pills that will prevent the major diseases of our time. Pop a pill and you can keep living that self-destructive lifestyle we call the American way of life. Unfortunately, it doesn't work that way and never will. "Lifestyle" is the key word because preventing (and reversing) diseases involves the interaction of many different factors and they can all be boiled down to how you live your life. And that can't be put in a pill.

At first glance, the RAVE Diet may sound like a negative, restrictive eating regimen, but nothing could be further from the truth. What it does is direct your eating habits away from heavily advertised, health-destructive foods and toward foods humans have eaten since the beginning. These foods have proven their success over eons in protecting humans from the diseases that have emerged as our biggest killers in just the last 100 years. These are clean-burning foods that will strengthen your entire body. The goal is to eliminate foods that interfere with or impair the body's defense systems, while increasing foods that strengthen the body's ability to heal itself.

You'll find you actually have a wide range of food choices "doin' the RAVE," and in the process you'll discover just how narrow your old eating habits actually were. In essence, what we're doing is eliminating the foods most people did not eat before the 20th century and most people throughout the world still do not eat today. It's an old-fashioned diet, but with some significant improvements. Think of it as an adventure not only in food, but also in health, that will have a profound payback over the years.

The RAVE Diet is uncompromising and strict adherence to it won't be possible for many. If that is the case for you, it should be thought of as an ideal diet – something to strive for – because the closer you follow it, the better the results. When followed to the letter, it works and works wonders.

The word RAVE is a simple acronym used to help people remember the rules. It is based on the guidelines used by doctors to treat and reverse diseases. This is what RAVE stands for:

No R efined foods
No A nimal foods
No V egetable oils
No E xceptions
   & Exercise

The following sections provide a succinct explanation.

No Refined Foods

"Unhealthy food is available everywhere all the time, like never before in history. Gas stations, drug stores, schools…" – Dr. Kelly D. Brownell, Yale University

"Hunters are using candy as bear bait. After gorging himself on candy, 'One bear just started walking around in circles…. Among the deleterious health effects: cavities, hair loss and lethargy.' If it does that to a 500 pound bear, just imagine what it does to humans." – Newsweek, November 3, 2003

Refined foods are plant foods that have been denatured and stripped of their fiber, vitamins, minerals, antioxidants and other nutrients. These foods are lifeless imitations of the vibrant products found in nature. They are devoid of any nutritional value and are usually transformed into dull, man-made foodstuffs that do not satisfy hunger, wreak havoc on your health and generally don't require teeth to eat them. Sadly, about *half* of the total calories in a typical American diet come from refined foods.

Refined foods are simple carbohydrates such as white flour, wheat flour, refined sugar, pastries, white pasta, white semolina, white bread, white rice, French fries, chips of any variety, cakes, soft drinks and similar junk foods. You know the foods I'm talking about – foods that have been transformed from their natural state into man-made products. (See *Reading Labels & Ingredients*.) This includes all refined soy- or rice-based meat and milk substitutes (e.g., soy/rice milk, tofu, etc). The only soy product allowed on this diet is the whole soy bean (endamame). The only rice product allowed is whole brown rice.

Because refined foods have no fiber, they spike your blood sugar, cause insulin surges, stimulate your appetite, accelerate the conversion of calories into body fat and promote many diseases. From your body's perspective, eating refined foods is, for all practical purposes, the same thing as eating refined sugar straight out of the box. From a weight loss perspective, refined foods do not fill you up, so you'll soon be hungry after eating them, which means you'll have to eat even more calories to feel full.

Many people think they are eating a plant-based diet because they are eating foods that do not contain animal products. Refined foods are every bit as bad for your body as animal foods and should be eliminated from your diet. A plant-based diet is about eating natural, whole plant foods. The health benefits of this diet (including weight loss) will be greatly diminished if refined foods are not eliminated from your diet.

Food manufacturers have spent billions of dollars researching ways to mix the right ingredients in order to "seduce" you into eating bad foods. Scientists have found that chocolate, for example, reaches its point of "maximum irresistibility" with a mix of 50 percent sugar and 50 percent fat.[1] But it doesn't stop there. Ingredient profiles have been created that are targeted down to genders and age groups in order to make refined foods as addicting as possible. If this reminds you of cigarette companies, you're thinking in the right direction.

Americans now spend about 90 percent of their food budget on refined foods. As a result of processing foods, the natural flavor is destroyed and has to be replaced with chemical additives. In fact, the heart of food flavor in America does not come from natural foods at all, but the refineries and chemical plants that dot an industrial corridor along the New Jersey turnpike.

Chemical flavoring not only accounts for the flavor in refined foods, but also in most of the meat Americans consume. Eric Schlosser documents this flavoring via chemistry with the following account:

> "After closing my eyes, I suddenly smelled a grilled hamburger. The aroma was uncanny, almost miraculous. It smelled like someone in the room was flipping burgers on a hot grill. But when I opened my eyes, there was just a narrow strip of white paper [under my nose] and a smiling flavorist."[2]

---

[1] Breaking the Food Seduction, Neal Barnard, M.D., p. 46.
[2] Fast Food Nation, Eric Schlosser, p. 129.

Ninety percent of the money Americans shell out for food buys a mix of chemistry and fiber-less, processed foodstuffs devoid of any real nutritional merit. This is how removed we have become from real food. We have not only lost our taste for real food, but we've come to prefer the taste of chemicals.

If that wasn't bad enough, 75 percent of all refined foods – from sodas to soups – contain genetically engineered ingredients.

As opposed to the *simple carbohydrates* found in refined foods, *complex carbohydrates* are found in natural, whole foods, such as whole grains, vegetables and fruits. These are the good carbohydrates that keep your blood sugar level on an even keel, promote health and keep you feeling full longer because they contain their natural fiber and all the nutrients nature gave them.

Always use *whole*-wheat pastas or *whole* wheat breads because they kept their fiber on the way to the grocery store. Make sure the label says whole wheat, *not* wheat flour. With grain products, the first ingredient should always have the word "whole" in it, sprouted wheat or organic rolled oats. Don't let the words "hearty wheat," "stoned wheat," or "multigrain" on the package fool you. This is just healthy-sounding advertising because these ingredients are made from refined white flour. And there is no difference between white flour and wheat flour. Wheat flour has some caramel coloring so it looks brown and sounds healthier, but it's the same as white flour.

Those who complain about carbohydrates are complaining about *refined*, or simple, carbohydrates, not the *complex* carbohydrates found in whole, natural foods. Those in pursuit of weight loss on "low-carb" diets are trading one set of problems for another because their diets are lacking in nutrients, particularly antioxidants, vitamins and minerals, which are essential for good health and can only be found in whole plant foods. (This is one reason why many low-carb diets recommend that people take supplements – in order to make up for the poor nutrition of such diets.)

Plant fiber does a number of miraculous things for your health, but one thing it does best is remove toxic substances from your body so you can flush them down the toilet. Fiber even removes heavy metals such as mercury, which you probably have in your body as a result of eating fish – or farm animals that were fed fishmeal. Fiber also removes cholesterol – the reason a fiber-rich diet will lower your cholesterol. In addition, fiber binds with sex hormones, such as estrogen, and removes them from your body. In the case of estrogen, American women have very high levels of estrogen due not only to our high-fat diet, but also due to the lack of fiber in our diets. Fiber also slows down glucose absorption and controls the rate of digestion, making food act more like a time-release pill, *which will keep you feeling full longer*.

Think of plant fiber as your intestinal broom because it will clean out a dirty bowel and prevent bad things from happening, like colon cancer. One of the major reasons refined foods and animal foods are not part of the RAVE Diet is because they do not contain fiber.

If you don't think you're eating much refined food now, I have a small experiment for you. All refined foods come in some kind of packaging. Every time you eat any refined food, keep the packaging it came in and put it in a bag. Do this for a week and at the end of the week inspect the contents of the bag. That should be enough to scare you into eliminating refined foods from your diet.

No Animal Foods

When we kill animals to eat them, they end up killing us because their flesh, which contains cholesterol and saturated fat, was never intended for human beings, who are natural herbivores. – William Clifford Roberts, M.D., Editor-in-Chief, American Journal of Cardiology

"No one can contemplate directly eating 13 pats of butter, but they essentially do when they eat a cheeseburger." – William Connor, M.D., The New American Diet

"Cancer is most frequent where carnivorous habits prevail." – Scientific American, 1892

All animal foods are excluded from the RAVE Diet because they promote the major degenerative diseases sweeping across the country. The link between animal foods and cancer, for example, begins back in 1892 with a study published in the *Scientific American* from which the quote above is taken. Subsequently, there has been a mountain of evidence compiled that confirms the link.[3]

---

[3] A small sampling: Skog KI, Johansson MAE, Jagerstad MI. Carcinogenic heterocyclic amines in model systems and cooked foods: a review on formation, occurrence, and intake. Food and Chem Toxicol 1998;36:879-96; Cummings JH, Bingham SA. Diet and the prevention of cancer. BMJ 1998;317:1636-40; Doll R, Peto R. The causes of cancer: quantitative estimates of avoidable risks of cancer in the United States today. J Natl Canc Inst 1981;66:1191-308; Kromhout D. Essential micronutrients in relation to carcinogenesis. Am J Clin Nutr 1987;45:1361-7; Munoz de Chavez M, Chavez A. Diet that prevents cancer: recommendations from the American Institute for Cancer Research. Int J Cancer Suppl 1998;11:85-9; Makinodan T, Lubinski J, Fong TC. Cellular, biochemical, and molecular basis of T-cell senescence. Arch Pathol Lab Med 1987;111:910-4; Chandra S, Chandra RK. Nutrition, immune response, and outcome. Progress in Food and Nutrition Science 1986;10:1-65; Barone J, Hebert JR, Reddy MM. Dietary fat and natural-killer cell activity. Am J Clin Nutr 1989;50:861-7; Nordenstrom J, Jarstrand C, Wiernik A. Decreased chemotactic and random migration of leukocytes during intralipid infusion. Am J Clin Nutr 1979;32:2416-22; Malter M, Schriever G, Eilber U. Natural killer cells, vitamins, and other brood components of vegetarian and omnivorous men. Nutr Cancer 1 989;12:271-8; Lauffer RB. Iron

46 - The RAVE Diet & Lifestyle

Balance. New York, NY: St. Martin's Press, 1991; Armstrong B, Doll R. Environmental factors and cancer incidence and mortality in different countries, with special reference to dietary practices. Int J Cancer 1975;15:617-31; Hirayama T. Epidemiology of breast cancer with special reference to the role of diet. Prev Med 1978;7:173-95; Lands WEM, Hamazaki T, Yamazaki K, et al. Changing dietary patterns. Am J Clin Nutr 1990;51:991-3; Carroll KK, Braden LM. Dietary fat and mammary carcinogenesis. Nutrition and Cancer 1985;6:254-9; Rose DP, Boyar AP, Wynder EL. International comparisons of mortality rates for cancer of the breast, ovary, prostate, and colon, and per capita food consumption. Cancer 1986;58:2363-71; U.S. Department of Health and Human Services. Surgeon General's Report on Nutrition and Health. DHHS Publ No. 88-50210, 1988; Rose DP, Boyar AP, Cohen C, Strong LE. Effect of a low-fat diet on hormone levels in women with cystic breast disease. 1. Serum steroids and gonadotropins. J Natl Cancer Inst 1987;78(4):623-6; Ingram DM, Bennett FC, Willcox D, de Klerk N. Effect of low-fat diet on female sex hormone levels. J Natl Cancer Inst 1987;79:1225-9; Goldin BR, Gorbach SL. Effect of diet on the plasma levels, metabolism and excretion of estrogens. Am J Clin Nutr 1988;48:787-90; Toniolo P, Riboli E, Protta F, Charrel M, Cappa AP. Calorie-providing nutrients and risk of breast cancer. J Natl Cancer Inst 1989;81:278; Robbana-Barnat S, Rabache M, Rialland E, Fradin J. Heterocyclic amines: occurrence and prevention in cooked food. Environ Health Perspect 1996;104:280-8; Thiebaud HP, Knize MG, Kuzmicky PA, Hsieh DP, Felton JS. Airborne mutagens produced by frying beef, pork, and a soy-based food. Food Chem Toxicol 1995;33(10):821-8; De Stefani E, Ronco A, Mendilaharsu M, Guidobono M, Deneo-Pellegrini H. Meat intake, heterocyclic amines, and risk of breast cancer: a case-control study in Uruguay. Cancer Epidemiol Biomarkers Prev 1997;6(8):573-81; Matos EL, Thomas DB, Sobel N, Vuoto D. Breast cancer in Argentina: case-control study with special reference to meat eating habits. Neoplasma 1991;38(3):357-66; Howe GR, Hirohata T, Hislop T, et al. Dietary factors and risk of breast cancer: combined analysis of 12 case-control studies. J Natl Cancer Inst 1990;82:561-9; Lubin F, Ruder AM, Wax Y, Modan B. Overweight and changes in weight throughout adult life in breast cancer etiology. Am J Epidemiol 1985;122:579-88; Elwood JM, Cole P, Rothman KJ, Kaplan SD. Epidemiology of endometrial cancer. J Natl Cancer Inst 1977;59:1055-60; Carter BS, Carter HB, Isaacs JT. Epidemiologic evidence regarding predisposing factors to prostate cancer. Prostate 1990;16:187-97; Howell MA. Factor analysis of international cancer mortality data and per capita food consumption. Br J Cancer 1974;29:328-36; Kolonel LN, Hankin JH, Lee J, Chu SY, Nomura AMY, Hinds MW. Nutrient intakes in relation to cancer incidence in Hawaii. Br J Cancer 1981;44:332-9; Rotkin ID. Studies in the epidemiology of prostatic cancer: expanded sampling. Cancer Treat Rep 1977;61:173-80; Schuman LM, Mandel JS, Radke A, Seal U, Halberg F. Some selected features of the epidemiology of prostatic cancer: Minneapolis-St. Paul, Minnesota case control study, 1976-1979. In: Magnus K, ed. Trends in Cancer Incidence: Causes and Practical Implications. Washington, DC: Hemisphere Publishing Corp., 1982; Graham S, Haughey B, Marshall J, et al. Diet in the epidemiology of carcinoma of the prostate gland. J Natl Cancer Inst 1983;70:687-92; Ross RK, Shimizu H, Paganini-Hill A, Honda G, Henderson BE. Case-control studies of prostate cancer in blacks and whites in Southern California. J Natl Cancer Inst 1987;78:869-74; Severson RK, Nomura AM, Grove JS, Stemmermann GN. A

The only thing you'll miss from eating animal foods is the saturated fat, cholesterol and animal proteins[4] – as well as the diseases these ingredients bring to your body. When you come right down to it, all our nutrients are ultimately obtained from plant foods. Meat-eating animals (including humans) feed off plant-eating animals, which really amount to storage systems for plant nutrients. The problem, of course, is that the plant nutrients in animals are delivered in a package of saturated fat and cholesterol. So why eat animals when you can get everything you need directly from plants – without the cholesterol – and in a low-fat package with healthy fiber and cancer-fighting chemicals to boot?

And calorie for calorie, plant foods are far richer in nutrients than animal foods, with green vegetables being the most nutrient-rich foods on the planet.

From a weight loss perspective, many studies have confirmed that over time, the more people eat meat, the more they gain weight. The more people eat whole

---

prospective study of demographics, diet, and prostate cancer among men of Japanese ancestry in Hawaii. Cancer Research 1989;49:1857-60; Oishi K, Okada K, Yoshida O, et al. A case control study of prostatic cancer with reference to dietary habits. Prostate 1988;12:179-90; Mettlin C, Selenskas S, Natarajan N, Huben R. Beta-carotene and animal fats and their relationship to prostate cancer risk: a case-control study. Cancer 1989;64:605-12; Hirayama T. Epidemiology of prostate cancer with special reference to the role of diet. Natl Cancer Inst Monogr 1979;53:149-54; Phillips RL. Role of lifestyle and dietary habits in risk of cancer among Seventh-day Adventists. Cancer Research 1975;35:3513-22; Mills P, Beeson WL, Phillips RL, Fraser GE. Cohort study of diet, lifestyle, and prostate cancer in Adventist men. Cancer 1989;64:598-604; Willett WC, Stampfer MJ, Colditz GA, Rosner BA, Speizer FE. Relation of meat, fat, and fiber intake to the risk of colon cancer in a prospective study among women. N Engl J Med 1990;323:1664-72; Gerhardsson de Verdier M, Hagman U, Peters RK, Steineck G, Overvik E. Meat, cooking methods, and colorectal cancer: a case-referrent study in Stockholm. Int J Cancer 1991;49:520-5; Singh PN, Fraser GE. Dietary risk factors for colon cancer in a low-risk population. Am J Epidemiol 1998;148(8):761-74; Giovannucci E, Rimm EB, Stampfer MJ, Colditz GA, Ascherio A, Willett WC. Intake of fat, meat, and fiber in relation to risk of colon cancer. Cancer Res 1994;54(9):2390-7; World Cancer Research Fund. Food, Nutrition, and the Prevention of Cancer: A Global Perspective. American Institute of Cancer Research. Washington, DC: 1997; Gregorio DI, Emrich LJ, Graham S, Marshall JR, Nemoto T. Dietary fat consumption and survival among women with breast cancer. J Natl Cancer Inst 1985;75:37-41; Verreault R, Brisson J, Deschenes L, Naud F, Meyer F, Belanger L. Dietary fat in relation to prognostic indicators in breast cancer. J Natl Cancer Inst 1988;80:819-25; Newman SC, Miller AB, Howe CR. A study of the effect of weight and dietary fat on breast cancer survival time. Am J Epidemiol 1986;123:767-74; Holm LE, Callmer E, Hjalmar ML, Lidbrink E, Nilsson B, Skoog L. Dietary habits and prognostic factors in breast cancer. J Natl Cancer Inst 1989;81:1218-23; Donegan WL, Hartz AJ, Rimm AA. The association of body weight with recurrent cancer of the breast. Cancer 1978;41:1590-4; Schapira DV, Kumar NB, Lyman GH, Cox CE. Obesity and body fat distribution and breast cancer prognosis. Cancer 1991;67:523-8.

[4] If you are worried about not getting enough protein, see *Notes – Protein*.

48 - The RAVE Diet & Lifestyle

plant foods, the less likely they are to gain weight. In a recent multi-nation study, it was found that *without exception,* the thinnest people ate a *complex carbohydrate* diet, while the fattest people ate a meat-based diet.[5] Eliminating meat from your diet is essential if you want to achieve your ideal weight, reverse heart disease and protect yourself against cancers and our major degenerative diseases.

From your heart's perspective, the difference between "lighter" meats and red meat is insignificant and much like the difference between regular cigarettes and "light" cigarettes. All meats – from red meat to chicken to turkey to fish to liquid meat (dairy) promote our major degenerative diseases.

The role of animal protein with respect to cancer deserves discussion. In the 1960s, researchers in India thought by increasing animal protein, it would actually help cure cancer. What they found was just the opposite. In 100 percent of the cases, increasing the consumption of animal protein *caused* cancer.[6] During the 1980s, Dr. Robert Good discovered that mice which were fed a low protein diet had fewer cancers. He followed this up by studying the low-protein diets of aborigines in Australia, who had extremely low rates of cancer.[7] Most recently, Dr. T. Colin Campbell[8] has also confirmed the animal protein-cancer connection, but with more precision and depth. Following the lead of the researchers in India, he injected rats with a powerful carcinogen (aflatoxin), to induce liver cancer.[9] When they were fed a 20 percent animal protein diet, *100 percent* of them developed cancer. When they were fed a five percent animal protein diet, *none* of them developed cancer, despite the presence of the

---

[5] Stable behaviors associated with adults' 10-year change in body mass index and likelihood of gain at the waist, H.S. Kahn, L.M. Tatham, C. Rodriguez, et al, Am. J. Public Health 87 (5): 747-57 and American Heart Association Annual Conference on Cardiovascular Disease Epidemiology and Prevention, San Francisco, 2004. American Heart Association news conference; participants: Robert H. Eckel, MD, University of Colorado Health Sciences Center; Randal J. Thomas, MD, Mayo Clinic, Rochester, Minn.; Deborah J. Toobert, PhD, Oregon Research Institute, Eugene, Ore.; Kristie J. Lancaster, PhD, RD, New York University, N.Y.; Alison Jane Rigby, PhD, MPH, RD, Stanford University, Palo Alto, Calif.; and Linda Van Horn, PhD, Northwestern University, Chicago.

[6] Madhavan TV, and Gopalan C., The effect of dietary protein on carcinogenesis of aflatoxin." Arch. Path. 85 (1968): 133-137.

[7] Good, Robert A., Fernandes, Gabriel, and Day, Noorbibi D., The Influence of Nutrition on Development of Cancer Immunity and Resistance to Mesenchymal Diseases, 1982, New York Raven Press, Molecular Interrelations of Nutrition and Cancer; A New Cancer Link:Gene-Pool Pollution," Modern Medicine, 11/29/71, p. 13; Diet Linked to Cancer Control, San Francisco Chronicle, 10/21/71.

[8] T. Colin Campbell, Ph.D. and Thomas M. Campbell II, The China Study.

[9] Dunaif, GE, Campbell TC, Dietary Protein level and aflatoxin B1-induced preneoplastic hepatic lesions in the rat. Nutrition 117 No. 7, 1987: 1298-302.

carcinogen. Dr. Campbell found that cancer could actually be turned on and off by simply changing the amount of animal protein in the diet.

In contrast, when the animals were fed a diet of 20 percent *vegetable* protein, *none of them developed cancer*, despite the presence of the carcinogen. Cancer was only triggered with animal protein, above a threshold of about eight percent of total calories. In further experiments, he found that regardless of how many carcinogens entered the body, the development of cancer was totally dependent on how much animal protein was consumed, *not the amount of carcinogens*. In other words, the animal protein served to "fertilize" the carcinogens and trigger the onset of cancer. In the absence of animal protein (or at very low levels), cancers were not triggered.

Dr. Campbell did his studies using dairy protein (casein), but he also investigated whether nutrients other than dairy protein might promote or reverse cancers. With stunning consistency, nutrients from *all animal foods grew tumors*, while nutrients from *all plant foods shrank tumors*.

In yet further tests, it was found that casein, the primary protein in all dairy products, was the most aggressive cancer promoter of all.[10]

How well do these laboratory studies translate into human terms? Dr. Campbell has two answers. The first is that although his studies were with rats, the biochemistry of cancer causation between rats and humans is the same.[11] Second, he directed the largest nutritional study ever conducted in human history, The China Project.[12] After detailed analysis of dietary patterns, down to the village level, he concluded that differences in cancer rates corresponded directly to differences in the amount of animal protein consumed: the more animal protein, the more cancer.

Another reason why animal protein causes cancer has to do with digestive enzymes – or a shortage of them as a result of eating animal foods.[13] Cancer cells have a protective protein coating around them which makes them *invisible* to the immune system. The pancreas produces two enzymes[14] that help digest animal protein. In addition to digesting animal protein, only these enzymes can dissolve the protein coating around cancer cells. Once the protein coating is dissolved by the enzymes, the cancer cells become *visible* and the immune system can do its job of destroying them.

---

[10] Inhibition of hepatocellular carcinoma development in hepatitis B virus transfected mice by low dietary casein, Cheng, Z, Hu, J., King, J., et al., Hepatology 26 No. 5 (1997: 1351-54).

[11] From an interview with T. Colin Campbell in the film, Healing Cancer From Inside Out by Mike Anderson.

[12] More information can be found at www.nutrition.cornell.edu/chinaproject/.

[13] This was first documented by Dr. John Beard in his book published in 1911, The Enzyme Treatment of Cancer And Its Scientific Basis. For more information, see the write up in Richard Walters, Options - The Alternative Cancer Therapy Book.

[14] Trypsin and chymotripsin.

Animal protein requires a lot of enzymes to digest it and eating a diet high in animal protein can cause a shortage of pancreatic enzymes. When this happens, cancer cells will keep their protective protein coating and remain invisible to the immune system – and start multiplying. The more animal protein you eat, in other words, the more you impair your body's natural defenses against cancer.

In contrast, pancreatic enzymes are not necessary to digest vegetable protein – so you can eat as much vegetable protein as you want and the supply of pancreatic enzymes available to unmask cancer cells will be remain plentiful.

Therapies based on pancreatic enzyme supplementation have been successful in treating cancer,[15] but it's much easier – and cheaper – to simply eliminate animal products from your diet.

These findings fit together with Dr. Campbell's findings: Animal protein promotes cancer and vegetable protein does not. In fact, vegetable protein does just the opposite: It fights cancer. These findings also agree with thousands of studies linking animal-based diets with cancer. What's amazing is that it has taken all these studies to confirm what was obvious to observers in the 1890s.

Cancer is very rare in areas of the world where people eat low-fat, plant-based diets. There is 120 times less incidence of prostate cancer, for example, in China compared to the United States.[16] As the Chinese change to the Western diet, however, their risk increases proportionally with their higher intake of animal foods.[17] This was demonstrated in a study in China where they found a man's chance for developing prostate cancer increased with the increased consumption of animal products.[18] Migration studies have also shown that as people leave their low-fat, plant-based diets behind and adopt the "standard American diet and lifestyle," their risk of cancer increases with each year of residence in their new country.[19]

With respect to some cancers, there is a little known problem with eating meat and dairy: 89 percent of the herds in the US are infected with the leukemia virus, which cause leukemia and lymphomas in cows.[20] This isn't just an American

---

[15] One of the main practitioners of this type of therapy is Dr. Nicolas Gonzales. For more information see www.dr-gonzalez.com/. For a recent news article on this see www.msnbc.msn.com/id/20164234/.

[16] Wang Y. Decreased growth of established human prostate LNCaP tumors in nude mice fed a low-fat diet. J Natl Cancer Inst. 1995 Oct 4;87(19):1456-62.

[17] Sung JF. Risk factors for prostate carcinoma in Taiwan: a case-control study in a Chinese population. Cancer. 1999 Aug 1;86(3):484-91.

[18] Lee MM. Case-control study of diet and prostate cancer in China. Cancer Causes Control. 1998 Dec;9(6):545-52.

[19] For example, see Whittemore AS. Prostate cancer in relation to diet, physical activity, and body size in blacks, whites, and Asians in the United States and Canada. J Natl Cancer Inst. 1995 May 3;87(9):652-61.

[20] Buehring GC, Philpott SM, Choi KY. Humans have antibodies reactive with Bovine leukemia virus. AIDS Res Hum Retroviruses. 2003 Dec;19(12):1105-13.

problem as 84% of herds in Argentina and 70% in Canada also have the bovine leukemia virus,[21] as well as high percentages in other meat-eating countries throughout the world. Some countries, such as Finland, have thoroughly eliminated the virus from their cattle, after some 30 years of effort.[22] In the study cited above, regarding American cattle, researchers found that 74 percent of the people they tested had been infected by this bovine virus, due to their meat- and dairy-based diets.

In addition to infecting white blood cells, these bovine viruses also attack other cells in the body, such as cells of the breast and the lymph nodes. One study found the virus in the breast tissues of 10 of 23 human breast cancer patients.[23]

In America and worldwide, leukemia and lymphoma are much more common in populations consuming higher amounts of dairy and beef,[24] particularly among dairy farmers,[25] while people working in occupations associated with cattle have twice the risk of developing leukemia and lymphoma.[26]

---

[21] Sargeant JM. Associations between farm management practices, productivity, and bovine leukemia virus infection in Ontario dairy herds. Prev Vet Med. 1997 Aug;31(3-4):211-21; VanLeeuwen JA,. Seroprevalence of infection with Mycobacterium avium subspecies paratuberculosis, bovine leukemia virus, and bovine viral diarrhea virus in maritime Canada dairy cattle. Can Vet J. 2001 Mar;42(3):193-8; Trono KG. Seroprevalence of bovine leukemia virus in dairy cattle in Argentina: comparison of sensitivity and specificity of different detection methods. Vet Microbiol. 2001 Nov 26;83(3):235-48.

[22] Nuotio L, Rusanen H, Sihvonen L, Neuvonen E. Eradication of enzootic bovine leukosis from Finland. Prev Vet Med. 2003 May 30;59(1-2):43-9.

[23] GC Buehring, KY Choi and HM Jensen. Bovine leukemia virus in human breast tissues. Breast Cancer Res 2001, 3(Suppl 1):A14; Buehring GC Evidence of bovine leukemia virus in human mammary epithelial cells Semin Cell Dev Biol 199735: 27A; Abstract V-1001.

[24] Sarasua S, Savitz DA. Cured and broiled meat consumption in relation to childhood cancer: Denver, Colorado (United States). Cancer Causes Control. 1994 Mar;5(2):141-8; Zhang S, Hunter DJ, Rosner BA, Colditz GA, Fuchs CS, Speizer FE, Willett WC. Dietary fat and protein in relation to risk of non-Hodgkin's lymphoma among women. J Natl Cancer Inst. 1999 Oct 20;91(20):1751-8; Fritschi L, Johnson KC, Kliewer EV, Fry R; Canadian Cancer Registries Epidemiology Research Group. Animal-related occupations and the risk of leukemia, myeloma, and non-Hodgkin's lymphoma in Canada. Cancer Causes Control. 2002 Aug;13(6):563-71; Chiu BC. Diet and risk of non-Hodgkin lymphoma in older women. JAMA. 1996 May 1;275(17):1315-21; Cunningham AS. Lymphomas and animal-protein consumption. Lancet. 1976 Nov 27;2(7996):1184-6.

[25] Hursting SD. Diet and human leukemia: an analysis of international data. Prev Med. 1993 May;22(3):409-22; Howell MA. Factor analysis of international cancer mortality data and per capita food consumption. Br J Cancer. 1974 Apr;29(4):328-36; Kristensen P. Incidence and risk factors of cancer among men and women in Norwegian agriculture. Scand J Work Environ Health. 1996 Feb;22(1):14-26; Reif J. Cancer risks in New Zealand farmers. Int J Epidemiol. 1989 Dec;18(4):768-74; Blair

Each year about 30,000 new cases of leukemia and 70,000 new cases of lymphoma occur for "unknown reasons" in the US, and undoubtedly many are caused by the bovine virus. The best way to protect yourself against this virus, is to avoid meat and dairy products and eat the RAVE way as it's been shown to greatly reduce your risk of being infected.[27]

So what about fish (or shellfish)[28]? No study has ever demonstrated that fish is heart-healthy.[29] The studies that have been done only show it mitigates the risk of sudden cardiac death among those already suffering heart disease – simply because it's a blood thinner and prevents clotting. This has been translated by the press into somehow preventing heart disease, but that is simply not true. The hype in the press regarding fish is about treating a symptom of heart disease (namely a heart attack) – and prolonging the disease – not preventing, arresting or reversing it. In fact, fish-based diets promote heart disease due to the high levels of cholesterol and saturated fat. Given that, it shouldn't be surprising that eating fish also causes a rise in blood cholesterol levels similar to the rise caused by beef and pork.[30]

Men with angina were advised to eat two portions of oily fish each week or take three fish oil capsules daily. They were found to have a higher risk of

---

A. Leukemia cell types and agricultural practices in Nebraska. Arch Environ Health. 1985 Jul-Aug;40(4):211-4; Donham KJ. Epidemiologic relationships of the bovine population and human leukemia in Iowa. Am J Epidemiol. 1980 Jul;112(1):80-92.

[26] Fritschi L, Johnson KC, Kliewer EV, Fry R; Canadian Cancer Registries Epidemiology Research Group. Animal-related occupations and the risk of leukemia, myeloma, and non-Hodgkin's lymphoma in Canada. Cancer Causes Control. 2002 Aug;13(6):563-71.

[27] Zhang SM, Hunter DJ, Rosner BA, Giovannucci EL, Colditz GA, Speizer FE, Willett WC. Intakes of fruits, vegetables, and related nutrients and the risk of non-Hodgkin's lymphoma among women. Cancer Epidemiol Biomarkers Prev. 2000 May;9(5):477-85; Marilyn L. Kwan, Gladys Block, Steve Selvin, Stacy Month, and Patricia A. Buffler. Food Consumption by Children and the Risk of Childhood Acute Leukemia. Am. J. Epidemiol. 2004 160: 1098-1107.

[28] Calorie for calorie, shell fish have high cholesterol levels, as well as high levels of saturated fat, and because they do not move around much, their toxic load is much higher than swimming fish. Some people think shell fish are somehow healthier, but they are not.

[29] Cundiff DK, Lanou AJ, Nigg CR. Relation of omega-3 Fatty Acid intake to other dietary factors known to reduce coronary heart disease risk. Am J Cardiol. 2007 May 1;99(9):1230-3. See also, Katan MB. Fish and heart disease: what is the real story? Nutr Rev 1995 Aug;53(8):228-30.

[30] Davidson MH, Hunninghake D, Maki KC, Kwiterovich PO Jr, Kafonek S. Comparison of the effects of lean red meat vs lean white meat on serum lipid levels among free-living persons with hypercholesterolemia: a long-term, randomized clinical trial. Arch Intern Med. 1999 Jun 28;159(12):1331-8.

cardiac death compared to men not given this advice.[31] Patients with coronary heart disease received fish oil capsules for some 28 months. It not only failed to lower their cholesterol, but their arteries closed even more during the study. The authors concluded: "Fish oil treatment for 2 years does not promote major favorable changes in the diameter of atherosclerotic coronary arteries."[32] A review of 48 randomized controlled trials involving over 36,000 participants who took fish oils or ate oily fish found no health benefits from these so-called "healthy fats." The conclusion: "Long chain and shorter chain omega 3 fats do not have a clear effect on total mortality, combined cardiovascular events, or cancer."[33] Men who consumed high levels of fish had a 60 percent increased risk of an acute coronary event and a nearly 70 percent increased risk of cardiovascular death, compared with men who consumed low amounts of fish.[34] In another study, men with high levels of mercury in their bodies had more than double the risk of a heart attack, compared to those with low levels.[35]

The contamination in fish is reason enough not to eat them. Fish and shellfish contain toxic chemicals at concentrations as high as 9 million times more than what was found in the polluted water in which they swam. Tests of fish from U.S. rivers have revealed they contained enough estrogen-mimicking chemicals to promote breast cancer growth,[36] not to mention the high levels of mercury, dioxins and PBCs that are found in fish and are highly associated with cancer and other diseases.

A survey of Lake Michigan fish found that 97 percent of the salmon and 91 percent of the lake trout were heavily contaminated with mercury and all of them were contaminated with PCBs.[37] Little wonder that children exposed to PCBs

---

[31] Burr ML, Ashfield-Watt PA, Dunstan FD, Fehily AM, Breay P, Ashton T, Zotos PC, Haboubi NA, Elwood PC. Lack of benefit of dietary advice to men with angina: results of a controlled trial. Eur J Clin Nutr. 2003 Feb;57(2):193-200.

[32] Sacks FM, Stone PH, Gibson CM, Silverman DI, Rosner B, Pasternak RC. Controlled trial of fish oil for regression of human coronary atherosclerosis. HARP Research Group. J Am Coll Cardiol. 1995 Jun;25(7):1492-8.

[33] Hooper L, Thompson RL, Harrison RA, Summerbell CD, Ness AR, Moore HJ, Worthington HV, Durrington PN, Higgins JP, Risks and benefits of omega 3 fats for mortality, cardiovascular disease, and cancer: systematic review. BMJ. 2006 Apr 1;332(7544):752-60.

[34] Jyrki K. Virtanen, et al. Mercury, Fish Oils, and Risk of Acute Coronary Events and Cardiovascular Disease, Coronary Heart Disease, and All-Cause Mortality in Men in Eastern Finland. Arterioscler. Thromb. Vasc. Biol., Jan 2005; 25: 228 - 233.

[35] Guallar E. Mercury, fish oils, and the risk of myocardial infarction. N Engl J Med. 2002 Nov 28;347(22):1747-54.

[36] Bringing Cancer to the Dinner Table: Breast Cancer Cells Grow Under Influence of Fish Flesh, Scientific American (online), April 17, 2007.

[37] EPA, Lake Michigan Mass Balance, 2004.

from Lake Michigan fish tend to have low IQs, poor reading comprehension, difficulty paying attention and memory problems.[38]

An actress who was eating tuna and other seafood four times a week, began experiencing severe headaches, cramping in her fingers and feet, and "...a sort of tingling, as if someone was tickling you, all up and down my body and on my legs, and it got more and more pronounced." She was unable to remember her lines, had crying spells, low-grade depression, loss of memory and brain fog.[39] She had, in fact, mercury poisoning from eating fish. Typical symptoms of mercury exposure include fatigue, headache, joint pain and reduced memory and concentration, but can include nervous system damage and even death.

A survey of over 23,000 postmenopausal women showed that fish consumption was positively associated with higher rates of breast cancer.[40] A number of other studies throughout the years have also shown that eating fish increases the risk of cancer, as well as the risk of the spread of cancer to other parts of the body.[41] In addition to the high fat levels of fish, fish oils also suppress the immune system.[42]

But even if there were "clean" fish available – and there are not – fish would still not be heart or cancer healthy due to the high levels of saturated fat, cholesterol, protein and the lack of fiber, complex carbohydrates and other vitamins.

When you look closely into the health claims of fish, they are in fact, very fishy. The original source of Omega-3 fats is plants and only plants can make Omega-3 fats. Why not get them from an uncontaminated source that is good for your health and perfectly balanced in terms of nutrients?

---

[38] Scott Fields, "Great lakes: resource at risk," Environmental Health Perspectives Vol. 113, No. 3 (March 2005), pgs. A164-A173. PCBs have also been linked to altering the sex ratio (the ratio of boys to girls born), reducing fertility, and causing abnormal menstrual cycles in women.

[39] Actress Describes Mercury Poisoning Ordeal, ABCNews, 10/21/05. www.abcnews.go.com/Health/story?id=1235251&page=1

[40] Connie Stripp, et al. Fish Intake Is Positively Associated with Breast Cancer Incidence Rate. J. Nutr. 133:3664-3669, November 2003.

[41] Griffini P. Dietary omega-3 polyunsaturated fatty acids promote colon carcinoma metastasis in rat liver. Cancer Res. 1998 Aug 1;58(15):3312-9; Klieveri L. Promotion of colon cancer metastases in rat liver by fish oil diet is not due to reduced stroma formation. Clin Exp Metastasis. 2000;18(5):371-7; Young MR. Effects of fish oil and corn oil diets on prostaglandin-dependent and myelopoiesis-associated immune suppressor mechanisms of mice bearing metastatic Lewis lung carcinoma tumors. Cancer Res. 1989 Apr 15;49(8):1931-6; Coulombe J. Influence of lipid diets on the number of metastases and ganglioside content of H59 variant tumors. Clin Exp Metastasis. 1997. Jul;15(4):410-7.

[42] Calder PC. Polyunsaturated fatty acids, inflammation, and immunity. Lipids. 2001;36:1007-24.

The one sure way we know that animal foods harm us is that our bodies start clearing out our arteries the minute we stop eating them. Dr. Nathan Pritikin, who pioneered heart disease reversal with diet, did not experience success in reversing his heart disease until he completely eliminated animal products from his diet.[43]

You do not need animal foods or "complete proteins" and you are much better off in all ways when you avoid them. You will also get more than enough protein on this diet. If you are concerned about protein issues, see *Notes – Protein* for more on this.

The protein requirement for normal adults is only two and a half percent of total calories. Mother's milk is five percent protein and that is at a time when the body is growing at its highest rate. More than five percent protein is not only unnecessary, but also potentially dangerous. Just one reason "high protein" diets should be avoided like the plague.

Bottom line: Animal foods cause disease. Not a single human being has ever failed to improve his or her health when he or she stopped eating animal foods. The evidence is simple, and simply overwhelming.

No Vegetable Oils

Strictly speaking, vegetable oils are part of the Refined Foods group because they contain no fiber, they're devoid of nutrients and they're 100 percent fat. Although I say vegetable oils, because these are what are mostly consumed, I mean *any oils* (e.g., nut oils, coconut oil, etc.).

Vegetable oils constitute a whopping 11 percent of the calories Americans consume.[44] Putting two tablespoons of oil in your salad has the fat equivalent of two scoops of ice cream. From a weight loss perspective, eliminating vegetable oils is a very easy – and healthy – way to cut calories. (See *Rave Diet Guidelines – Cooking Without Oil*.)

There are other problems with vegetable oils, however. These oils contain high levels of saturated fat, which is essentially "cholesterol in disguise" because it stimulates your liver to make more cholesterol than your body needs and ends up clogging arteries. In fact, adding *any* oil to your food will raise your cholesterol level, even more than eating cholesterol itself.[45]

Hydrogenated vegetable oils (trans-fats) are particularly efficient at clogging arteries and depriving your body of oxygen. These oils are found in all kinds of refined foods such as chips, cookies, crackers, cereals, breakfast bars and other

---

[43] The Pritikin Program for Diet & Exercise, Nathan Pritikin, M.D., p. 93. See also, the film *Eating* by Mike Anderson for other accounts.

[44] Eat To Live, Joel Fuhrman, M.D., p. 91.

[45] Dr. Dean Ornish's Program for Reversing Heart Disease, Dean Ornish, M.D., p. 256-257.

baked goods. Every time you eat a bag of cookies it's no different than biting into a piece of meat.

In packaged goods, look for the word "hydrogenated" in the ingredients list and put it back on the shelf. And any food that's deep-fried, such as fast food French fries or donuts, will contain these artery-clogging oils. Many commercial brands of peanut butter will also use hydrogenated oils. If you like nut butters, grind your own at a health food store.

Hydrogenated oils are the "glue" that holds refined carbohydrates together in order to increase shelf life. In fact, the healthy amount of trans fats in your diet should be exactly zero. Ingredients used for longer shelf lives in food translate into longer illnesses and a shorter shelf life for you.

Fried animal foods, such as fried chicken, are probably the *most dangerous foods in existence* because they combine high levels of saturated fat and cholesterol, with high levels of oil. In other words, your blood vessels are getting a triple-whammy when you eat fried animal foods.

Even seemingly "innocent" foods such as movie popcorn are dangerous as they are usually popped in coconut or palm oil, both of which are extremely high in saturated fat.

The current rage among some health authorities is olive oil. It's ironic that our health authorities are advising an overweight nation to eat the most concentrated form of fat on the planet, which packs more calories, pound-for-pound, than butter. The basic reason (presumably) is that they are trying to move people away from margarine, although these same authorities (e.g., The American Heart Association and virtually all major health experts) were praising margarine just a few decades ago – and quoting studies purporting to show margarine, containing hydrogenated oils, was heart-healthy!

Although olive oil is healthier than butter or margarine, that's not saying much. It's probably the worst way to get heart-healthy fats because there's almost no nutritional bang for the calorie buck. In fact, olive and other oils are so nutritionally bankrupt that Joel Fuhrman, M.D., gives oils a score of 1 out of 100, just above refined sweets, which score a zero.[46]

Olive oil is 100 percent fat and contains high concentrations of saturated fat, while the fiber, antioxidants, vitamins and minerals of the olive itself have been stripped away. In clinical studies on humans, olive oil has been shown to be as bad for the heart as eating roast beef.[47] In other studies, it has been found that monounsaturated fat, although showing higher HDL and lower LDL levels, resulted in just as much coronary disease as saturated fat.[48]

---

[46] Eat To Live, Joel Fuhrman, M.D., p. 121.

[47] The Influence of Diet on the Appearance of New Lesions in Human Coronary Arteries, JAMA, 1990, Vol. 263, pp. 1646-52.

[48] Lawrence L. Rudel, et al., Arteriosclerosis, Thrombosis, and Vascular Biology, December, 1995; R. Vogel, et al., Journal of the American College of Cardiology,

Using the brachial artery tourniquet test, it was found that olive oil constricted blood flow by a whopping 31 percent![49] Why is this important? Because when arteries constrict, the endothelium (artery's lining) is injured, triggering plaque build-up or arthrosclerosis (heart disease).[50]

In addition, the Omega-3's in vegetable oils are highly unstable and tend to decompose and unleash free radicals that cause damage to cells. Vegetable oils have also been implicated in several different studies with cancers and polyunsaturated fat turn out to be the strongest promoter of skin cancers of all the foodstuffs we eat.[51] Vegetable oils also suppress the immune system and actually promote the spread of some cancers.[52]

Simply put, olive and other oils are bankrupt foods that have little nutritional value, a very high caloric cost and actually do damage to your body. If you're after the good fat in olives, get it from the olives themselves, not the denatured oil.

Some highly questionable studies[53] claim to show a "slower progression" of heart disease when people consume olive oil. But having a slower progression of heart disease hardly makes the case that olive oil is heart-healthy, assuming such a causal relationship exists in the first place. Other studies have shown it is not the olive oil at all, but the high fiber content in a traditional Mediterranean-type diet that accounts for lower rates of heart disease.[54] A diet is not heart-healthy unless it arrests and reverses heart disease and only a whole, plant-based diet –

2000: The Postprandial Effect of Components of the Mediterranean Diet on Endothelial Function.

[49] Vogel RA. Corretti MC. Plotnick GD. The postprandial effect of components of the Mediterranean diet on endothelial function. Journal of the American College of Cardiology. 36(5):1455-60, 2000 Nov 1.

[50] High fat meals block the endothelium's ability to produce nitric oxide, which is a vasodilator and critical to preserving the tone and health of blood vessels. Moreover, fat should be released into the blood stream slowly and you can only get that slow release by eating natural plant foods in their natural packages that still contain their fiber.

[51] Harris RB, Foote JA, Hakim IA, Bronson DL, Alberts DS. Fatty acid composition of red blood cell membranes and risk of squamous cell carcinoma of the skin. Cancer Epidemiol Biomarkers Prev. 2005 Apr;14(4):906-12. See also John A. McDougall, M.D., www.drmcdougall.com/vegetable_fat.html.

[52] Young MR. Effects of fish oil and corn oil diets on prostaglandin-dependent and myelopoiesis-associated immune suppressor mechanisms of mice bearing metastatic Lewis lung carcinoma tumors. Cancer Res. 1989 Apr 15;49(8):1931-6; Coulombe J. Influence of lipid diets on the number of metastases and ganglioside content of H59 variant tumors. Clin Exp Metastasis. 1997 Jul;15(4):410-7.

[53] For example, the Lyon Diet Heart Study. Note that after nearly four years into the study, 25 percent of the subjects following the "heart-healthy" Mediterranean diet had either died or experienced some new cardiovascular event.

[54] European Journal of Clinical Nutrition 2002;56:715-722.

which specifically excludes *all* oils – has been proven to do that. Adding oils to such a diet only impairs its effectiveness.

The model for the Mediterranean diet harks back to the 1950's and before when people, especially in the island of Crete, were virtually free of heart disease – despite their indulgence in olive oil. This was not because of the olive oil, but because they ate primarily vegetables and whole grains, a little fish and got lots of exercise. Today, their consumption of olive oil has remained the same (if not increased), but their consumption of whole plant foods has plummeted, as has their exercise. As a result, heart disease and obesity have skyrocketed. [55] Olive oil has nothing to do with preventing heart disease and clinical studies have shown that it actually promotes arterial lesions.[56] It's just another magic bullet that is a big, fat fantasy promoted by the olive oil industry determined to get high levels of fat back into our diets.

When T. Colin Campbell, author of *The China Study*, was asked what the difference was between the Mediterranean diet and diets in rural China, where heart disease is practically nonexistent, he replied "I would say the absence of oil in the rural Chinese diet is the reason for their superior success."[57]

The leading health authorities in reversing heart disease with diet, including Dr. Caldwell Esselstyn, Dr. Joel Fuhrman, Dr. John McDougall and Dr. Dean Ornish, all agree that vegetable oils should be *excluded* from a heart-healthy diet. These doctors actually reverse heart disease as opposed to those who just talk about it or promote the greasy stuff because of financial ties to the olive oil industry. In fact, there has not been a single case of heart disease arrest or reversal where any vegetable oil was a part of the diet. So, if olive oil is so "heart-healthy," why would doctors who reverse heart disease specifically exclude it? Because they consider vegetable oils to be "heart dangerous" and so should you.

In a nutshell, here's the argument against oils: *all* dietary fats – be they animal or plant fats of all kinds – at levels above 20 percent of total calories, cause heart disease. This has been demonstrated in many clinical tests.[58] In order to prevent

---

[55] The same sort of argument is made by those peddling any oil. Coconut oil vendors, for example, will argue that despite its very high saturated fat content, populations consuming large quantities of coconut products (such as in the Philippines), have low rates of heart disease. Again, this is due to their overall (traditional) low fat, low cholesterol diet. The low rates of heart disease were achieved not because of the coconut oil, but despite it.

[56] The Influence of Diet on the Appearance of New Lesions in Human Coronary Arteries, JAMA, 1990, Vol. 263, pp. 1646-52.

[57] During a panel discussion at the 2nd National Summit on Cholesterol and Coronary Artery Disease, as quoted in Prevent and Reverse Heart Disease, Caldwell B. Esselstyn, M.D., p. 84.

[58] The Influence of Diet on the Appearance of New Lesions in Human Coronary Arteries," D. H. Blankenhorn; R. L. Johnson; W. J. Mack; H. A. el Zein; L. I. Vailas,

heart disease, you have to reduce your *overall* fat intake. A diet of 100 percent whole plant foods is as heart-healthy as you can get. Why introduce a highly concentrated form of fat, such as vegetable oil, that will surely bring your fat intake level into an unsafe zone?

Oils should be put in vehicles and machinery, not your body. In fact, the original use of Canola oil was to lubricate machinery. Then someone came up with the bright idea that people might actually eat it. Flaxseed oil is commonly used as a thinner in paints and varnishes and when consumed in high quantities, can hamper the blood's ability to clot.

Instead of using vegetable oils for cooking, cook at lower temperatures and use water to make your own broth – or use the substitutes below. You'll be surprised at how well they work. And with a little practice, you'll soon find you prefer the cleaner taste. It's like the difference between eating peaches in heavy syrup and eating fresh peaches right off the tree. Once you stop using oils, you will be able to taste the difference and you'll never go back.

Oil substitutes for sautéing: apple juice, sherry, vegetable stock, vinegars, wine, beer

Oil substitutes in baked goods: applesauce, pureed bananas, pureed stewed prunes

---

JAMA, 1990, Vol. 263, pp. 1646-52; Lancet 344:1195, 1994); Aterioscler Thromb Vasc Biol 15:2101, 1995; Dietary Monounsaturated Fatty Acids Promote Aortic Atherosclerosis in LDL Receptor–Null, Human ApoB100–Overexpressing Transgenic Mice, Lawrence L. Rudel, Kathryn Kelley, Janet K. Sawyer, Ramesh Shah, Martha D. Wilson, Arterioscler Thromb Vasc Biol. 1998;18:1818-1827; Combined Intense Lifestyle and Pharmacologic Lipid Treatment Further Reduce Coronary Events and Myocardial Perfusion Abnormalities Compared With Usual-Care Cholesterol-Lowering Drugs in Coronary Artery Disease, Stefano Sdringola, MD, FACC, Keiichi Nakagawa, MD, Yuko Nakagawa, MD, S. Wamique Yusuf, MBBS, MRCP, Fernando Boccalandro, MD, Nizar Mullani, BS, Mary Haynie, RN, MBA, Mary Jane Hess, RN, K. Lance Gould, MD, FACC, Journal of the American College of Cardiology, JACC Vol. 41, No. 2, 2003, 263–72; Effect of Diet on Vascular Reactivity: An Emerging Marker for Vascular Risk, Sheila G. West, Current Atherosclerosis Reports, Vol 3.6, pp. 446-455; Effect of a High-Fat Ketogenic Diet on Plasma Levels of Lipids, Lipoproteins, and Apolipoproteins in Children, Peter O. Kwiterovich, Jr; Eileen P. G. Vining; Paula Pyzik; Richard Skolasky, Jr; John M. Freeman, JAMA. 2003;290:912-920; Rudel LL, Parks JS, Sawyer JK. Compared with dietary monounsaturated and saturated fat, polyunsaturated fat protects African Green Monkeys from coronary artery atherosclerosis. Arterioscler Thromb Vasc Biol 1995;15:2101- 2110; de Lorgeril M, Salen P, Martin JL, Monjaud I, Deloye J, Mamelle N. Mediterranean diet, traditional risk factors, and the rate of cardiovascular complications after myocardial infarction. Circulation 1999;99:779-785.

For salads, choose a dressing without oil or a vinegar-based dressing, such as a Balsamic or brown-rice-seasoned vinegar dressing. Or try citrus juices in place of salad dressing. If you don't like the taste of vinegar dressings, try mixing them with a tomato-based sauce to make your dressing. (See *Rave Diet Guidelines – Salad Dressings Without Oil.*) Many people have started off with this diet and could not stand the taste of vinegar – but now prefer it because their tastes have changed. Your tastes will change, too, if you give this a chance.

No Exceptions

"We all agree your theory is crazy, but is it crazy enough?" Niels Bohr, Nobel Laureate

Now, after all these negative "No's", you're probably thinking I'm crazy for also saying "No Exceptions" because everyone is going to have some exceptions in our world of plentiful temptations. That, however, is precisely why I say it. It's right out of the school of if you give them an inch, they'll take a mile.

If you are simply trying to lose weight, as opposed to reversing a disease, then I would say you could apply a "99 percent" RAVE rule, that is, follow the RAVE Diet for 99 percent of your caloric intake. In practical terms, this means having rare exceptions to these rules. Roger Ebert, the film critic, lost 89 pounds and described rare exceptions like this,

> "I agree with McDonald's that a visit to Mickey D's can be part of a responsible nutritional approach. That's why I've dined there twice in the last 17 months."[59]

In other words, if you follow Roger Ebert's example and dine at McDonald's every eight months or so, it won't set your weight goals back very much.

If you are fighting a disease, however, the No Exceptions rule should be applied to the letter. In fact, Dr. Nathan Pritikin followed a strict RAVE Diet when he reversed his heart disease, but subsequent book versions of his diet have made exceptions to his diet. If you want to prevent or reverse heart disease and the diseases associated with narrowing and closure of the blood vessels throughout your body, you will want to follow the RAVE Diet strictly – or it simply won't work. In fact, success on health issues will correspond directly with how strictly you follow the diet.

Doctors who administer dietary treatments to cure diseases will tell you the No Exception rule is the biggest area of concern. When patients stray from their diets, even a little, it can significantly undermine the goals they are trying to

---

[59] Supersize Me, Roger Ebert, Chicago Sun-Times, 5/7/04.

achieve. A friend of mine cured an arthritic knee by following the diet, but over the Christmas holidays he indulged – and the pain in his knee returned.

I can always tell when someone is not following the diet strictly – they don't lose weight. People who follow this diet without exceptions will lose weight, if they need to. When someone says to me, "The diet isn't working! I'm not losing weight!" I always volunteer to make an inspection of what's in their refrigerators and pantries – and they *always* say NO! That's because their kitchens are full of exceptions – and so too is their diet.

The RAVE Diet is the diet that not only prevents, but has also reversed heart and other diseases. Just eating a little more fruits, vegetables and whole grains won't do much, if anything, for your health. If you want to have a big impact, you have to make big changes.

I'm not a disciplinarian and I think that an occasional indulgence is fine – so long as it is very occasional. For example, you might have a piece of cake during a birthday party or you might indulge in small ways during holiday festivities. This is Ok, so long as you get right back into the RAVE Diet. The biggest problem is that occasional exceptions can easily lead you back into old habits.

Most of us think we can get away with more than just an occasional exception, but there is real pain involved in these exceptions. "Oh, these are only calories," you say. Ah, but they're not. They're usually *empty* calories, which means you'll soon be hungry again and you'll need to consume even more calories in order to feel full.

"So what?" you say. "I'll just work off the calories." Well, first of all, it's a lot easier to say you're going to work them off than it is to actually work them off. To work off a Snickers candy bar, you'd have to spend 51 minutes jogging or two hours walking just to get back where you were *before* you had a few minutes of pleasure eating that candy bar. A 20-ounce Coke will cost you nearly an hour of biking. In other words, these brief moments of pleasure can be very painful over the long run. (To think of it another way, you'd have to eat about three pounds of apples to equal the calories you consume in one five-ounce chocolate bar.)

Second, you can't "work off" cholesterol. The average person can only get rid of 100 mg of cholesterol a day. A single egg contains 213 mg and that excess cholesterol ends up clogging arteries. The only way you're going to get rid of cholesterol is to stop eating it and lower your saturated fat intake so you'll give your body a fighting chance to get rid of the excess. The body is extremely fine-tuned to handle this, but it can't function properly when it's overwhelmed.

You might think of the RAVE Diet as your lifelong marriage partner. You might have an occasional fling with Mr. Sweet or Ms. Fat or Mr. Salt, but these are temporary distractions that can't possibly give you a lifetime of satisfaction and love like the one your marriage partner can. The best advice I can give you is to stay faithful and monogamous and, like a good marriage, the payoffs will be incalculable.

Finally, your friends may laugh at you for following such a "crazy" diet. But they'll stop laughing when they see your new body and lifestyle. When they're suffering through the anguish of diet-related diseases later in life and you continue to dodge those disease-laden bullets, trust me, you'll have the last, crazy laugh.

Exercise

"The sovereign invigorator of the body is exercise, and of all exercises, walking is the best." – Thomas Jefferson

It always amazes me that we don't have half an hour to exercise, but manage to squeeze in an average of four hours of TV a day.

"What, are they allergic to sweat?" – Richard Simmons, fitness personality

Animals in the wild never get fat. Humans in the wild never get fat. Domesticate dogs, they get fat and diseased. Domesticate humans, they get fat and diseased. Our sedentary lifestyles are simply not suited to our Stone Age bodies.

Exercise is an essential part of the RAVE Diet. As mentioned previously, the root of the word diet actually means "lifestyle" and a change in diet really means a change in the style of your life. Active Americans get a fraction of the cancers and other diseases that sedentary Americans get. Among other things, exercise helps to correct bad health habits by burning up and stabilizing blood sugar levels, improving immune function and lymph flow, getting oxygen to all parts of the body and strengthening bones, while helping us handle stress and increasing both the quality and quantity of sleep.

Exercise also speeds the passage of carcinogens and toxins from the body and recent studies have shown that exercise keeps your brain as fit as your body, particularly as you age. In other words, exercise will not only make you feel fit and improve your appearance, but it will prevent a wide range of diseases.

As your main exercise, choose a regimen that's just the opposite of cancer – one that's aerobic – an exercise that makes you breathe and respire to raise the oxygen levels in your blood. Cancer hates oxygen and thrives in areas of your body with low oxygen levels, where the blood supply is limited, due to clogged blood vessels. It's no accident that the American Cancer Society recently made exercise a cornerstone of cancer prevention.

Walking is probably the best exercise for all of us. It's easy, cheap and gets you outdoors, which can do wonders for your mental state. It wasn't that long ago that walking wasn't an exercise at all, but transportation for the vast majority of Americans, so try to find opportunities during the day that allows you to walk more, instead of driving to a destination.

Always get at least half an hour of exercise a day, or 45 minutes five times a week. If you've had a busy day, even 15 minutes can be beneficial. Try walking for 30 minutes in the morning and 30 minutes in the evening. I guarantee it will transform your life within a month.

Get out in the sun occasionally. It will bring some perspective into your life, it's the best way to get vitamin D and recent studies have shown that moderate exposure has a protective effect against all sorts of cancers – including skin cancer. Just the opposite of what we've been told for the last 20 years.

And when the brain is producing "happy chemicals" – such those released when you exercise – they actually strengthen your immune system.

The best time to exercise is whenever you can, but most people prefer to exercise in the mornings because it seems to jump-start their metabolism, giving them more energy and mental acuity throughout the day. It's also easier to find the time in the early hours because there are usually fewer demands on your schedule.

Insofar as weight loss is concerned, exercise will reduce fat and build lean muscle mass, which will *increase your metabolism* and that, in turn, will burn more calories. The more exercise you get, the more muscle you gain. The more muscle you gain, the more your metabolism and energy will increase – and the more fat you'll burn.

When you're sedentary, you lose muscle mass. When active, you gain it and that is the key to burning more calories. Don't use the excuse that your metabolism slows down with age. Nonsense. Metabolism is a function of lean body mass, the more you have the higher your metabolism. Get moving, build up your lean body mass and your metabolism will move with you.

There's a secret known to those who exercise regularly: Exercise *creates* energy. Don't wait for energy to come to you when you're tired. When you feel that afternoon slump, shake it off and get your body moving. Taking a 15-minute walk will keep you more awake and alert the rest of the day than an afternoon nap – or that cup of coffee.

Humans are naturally lazy because we're programmed to conserve energy. In the past, we were forced to exercise to find food and there was a balance between the calories expended to locate or farm food and the calories we consumed. Today, we have created an incredibly artificial living environment that's also designed to conserve energy. The result is that many Americans are so inactive they're practically living their lives in bed rest! Humans in industrialized countries are very much like caged birds, but in our case we're caged in our chairs and couches. Despite our technical advances, we're still trapped in Stone Age bodies and those bodies need to be exercised – just as faithfully as they are fed every day.

The best incentive to exercise is that it simply makes you feel wonderful and alive! But if you need an immediate reason to exercise, here's one you can't resist – you'll enjoy a much better sex life! (For more, see *Sex, Booze, Rock 'n Roll*)

Essential Dietary Guidelines

Here are a few simple keys to the RAVE Diet.

The #1 Golden Rule: Always eat foods as close to their natural state as possible. Eat whole foods that come in their natural packages and avoid foods that come in a package or can, unless they are fresh-frozen. Some of the sample menus will contain items that are canned. This is for convenience. If you can find the item in its natural state or are willing to take the time to prepare it, instead of buying it in a can, then you should do so.

Always eat whole foods: In packaged goods, look for the words "whole," "sprouted wheat" or "organic rolled oats" in the first ingredient, not the second or third. Always eat whole-wheat pastas or whole wheat breads. Make sure the label says whole wheat, not wheat flour. Don't let the words "hearty wheat," "stoned wheat," or "multigrain" on the package fool you. Such ingredients are made from refined white flour and there's *no difference between white flour and wheat flour*. Wheat flour has some caramel coloring and sounds healthier, but it's not.

Eat a wide variety of colorful foods: Always eat a wide variety of foods because each food has its own special health benefits and disease fighting profiles – and they work as a team, complimenting, reinforcing and magnifying each other's benefits. This is the new math of cancer prevention and eating a variety of foods actually multiplies cancer-fighting and cardiovascular benefits because they work together synergistically. Along the same lines, most of the antioxidant benefits of fruits and vegetables come from the component that gives them their color, so make sure your plate is full of different colors – *the deeper and darker the colors, the more cancer-fighting nutrients*. The magic is in variety. Get in the habit of chopping up vegetables and putting them in containers, or buying vegetables already chopped up. That way, you can add a variety of foods to your meal very conveniently.

Uncooked Food: *Eat at least half of your food uncooked.* The more uncooked food, the better. In general, cooked or processed foods contain fewer phytochemicals and antioxidants than fresh and uncooked foods.[60] Some nutrients become bio-available only when you cook food, while others are only available in the food's uncooked state. (For more on this, see *Notes, Raw vs. Cooked Foods*.) Broccoli and other cruciferous vegetables such as cabbage, kale, Brussels sprouts, radishes, and cauliflower are the best sources of a powerful anti-cancer nutrient called sulforaphane. In human tests, the absorption rate of this compound was ten times higher in uncooked broccoli versus cooked broccoli.[61] Steaming is the best way to cook vegetables. Try to eat your food plain or with herbs and spices. If you buy good-tasting products in the first place, you won't need anything on them. Include lots of sprouted grains as a regular part of your meals.

A Salad Is An Ideal Meal: A salad puts into practice the previous four tips about eating. If you find that a salad takes too much time to prepare, simply stop by your local salad bar, be it in a restaurant or supermarket – but bring your own salad dressing, or use vinegar without oil. If you use sliced beets, the juice from them can serve as a delicious dressing.

Chew your food thoroughly: The idea behind reversing diseases with nutrition is to give your body a concentrated boost of nutrients. Key to this is the ability to fully digest the foods you are eating, in order to get the most nutrients from them. This is where enzymes come into play because enzymes help your body fully digest food. The first step you can take to increase enzyme activity is to chew food very thoroughly because the saliva in your mouth contains enzymes that will break down food and make it more digestible. A good rule of thumb is that your food should be close to liquid before you swallow it, i.e., you should "drink your food." The next place you can get enzymes is by eating uncooked foods. When food is cooked, digestive enzymes are destroyed and so, too, is the ability to get the most nutrients from foods. Eating raw, uncooked food retains the natural enzymes in foods and thus your ability to fully absorb their nutrients. It's for this one reason that we say to eat at least half of your food uncooked (above).

Never cook with salt: Natural plant foods contain all the sodium you'll ever need. People like to say that salt brings out the flavor in food. Nonsense! All it does is give food a salty taste and camouflage the real taste of food, while promoting blood clotting and high blood pressure. Learn to use spices and herbs, instead of salt, to flavor your food. Or try Mrs. Dash or Salt-Free Spike. A few weeks after you stop using salt, you'll find you won't miss it at all.

---

[60] Henry C, Heppell N (2002). "Nutritional losses and gains during processing: future problems and issues". Proc Nutr Soc 61 (1): 145–8.
[61] Suzanne Dixon, MPH, MS, RD. J Agric Food Chem 2008;56:10505-9.

Take a Multivitamin or B-12 Supplement: This is part of the standard RAVE Diet, as well. Some people think that having to take a supplement on what is supposedly an "all-natural" diet means it is deficient in some respect, but the opposite is actually the truth. B-12 is a vitamin that is synthesized by bacteria that live in the soil. It does not come from animals. Herbivorous animals happen to have B-12 because they consume soil when they eat plants, thereby storing B-12 in their flesh. Getting enough B-12 was never a problem for our ancestors because they came into contact with the soil constantly. It is only because our environment is so sanitary and our contact with the earth so infrequent that we require this supplement.

Get Adequate Amounts of Vitamin D: If there is a single micronutrient that practically all Americans are deficient in it is vitamin D, known as the "sunshine" vitamin. The best way to get this vitamin is through exposure to the sun. If you are not able to do this on a regular basis, take a daily vitamin D supplement of 1,000 IU. For additional details, see *Notes – Vitamin D*.

Ground Flaxseed: A teaspoon of ground flaxseed should be a part of your daily diet. Flaxseed is not only the single best source of fiber in the world, but it has been proven to be very effective in fighting breast cancer and, presumably, other hormone-based cancers such as prostate cancer. In one study, women eating flaxseed muffins every day proved that flaxseed was just as effective as Tamoxifen in shrinking cancer tumors – and without the side effects of an extremely toxic drug.[62] You can purchase a flaxseed grinder (coffee grinders work just as well) and store the ground seed in the refrigerator for up to two weeks. Any excess ground seed should be stored in the freezer to prevent the essential fatty acids (Omega-3's) from becoming rancid. Sprinkle it over anything and everything, from fruits to salads and oatmeal or any other dish. Avoid flaxseed oil, as it's a refined product and part of the restricted vegetable oil group in the RAVE Diet. (See *The RAVE Diet & Lifestyle – No Vegetable Oils*.)

Snacking: Snacking in-between meals is not bad in and of itself. It all depends on what you eat. Avoid packaged "snack" foods like the plague. Always eat whole plant foods, such as fruit or vegetables. Fruits are the best snack. The high concentration of water and fiber makes them very filling. If you are at work, bring an extra large helping of lunch and snack on that. (See *Fast Food: Meals In Minutes* for quick meal suggestions and *What To Expect* for more on snacking)

---

[62] Biological Effects of Dietary Flaxseed In Patients With Breast Cancer, Thompson LU, Li T, Chen J, Goss PE Nutritional Sciences, University of Toronto, Toronto, ON, Canada; Medical Oncology, Princess Margaret Hospital, Toronto, ON, Canada, San Antonio Breast Cancer Symposium 2000.

Beverages: Pure water should <u>always</u> be your beverage of choice. Any beverage containing any kind of sweetener is off limits. (See *Reading Labels & Ingredients*.) Any beverage containing a stimulant, such as caffeine, should be avoided, as well. Stimulants give you an "artificial" high because when you come down from them, you're at a lower point than you would have been without having taken them in the first place – the reason you need that second cup of coffee. Fruit juices are fine so long as they are unsweetened and contain the fiber or pulp from the whole fruit. There are no specific rules about fluid intake, except that you should drink as much water as you're comfortable with. If you're trying to lose weight, see the next section, *Accelerating Weight Loss,* for additional guidelines on water consumption. Avoid "sport drinks" and any drink that carries a "health" label with it. You're simply wasting your money. Alcohol should be avoided as much as possible. For cancer patients, drinking alcohol is particularly dangerous not only because of the high sugar content, which feeds cancer cells, but because it fuels the production of a growth factor that helps create new blood vessels inside tumors (angiogenesis), which will carry more fuel (glucose) to tumor cells.[63]

Eating Out: Ethnic restaurants usually have the best food choices, but in any restaurant, just order whatever is on the menu, but ask them to leave out the bad stuff by following the RAVE Diet rules. Simply say you don't eat meat and dairy and ask them to prepare a vegetable plate for you. You can request they not cook it in oil, but American chefs simply don't know how to do that. Steamed vegetables are the best and most restaurants can do this. Look at what they are offering as side dishes and ask that they make a special plate of side dishes for you. Stay away from restaurant pasta. Whole-wheat pasta is rare in restaurants and they all cook pasta with oil. If you're at a steak house, go for the baked potato and vegetable side dishes. Or head straight for the salad bar. When eating at a sushi bar, just order the vegetarian sushi. If it's not on the menu, just request it. Ask for Balsamic vinaigrette to dip your bread in, instead of oil. Better yet, ask for a plate of vegetables, instead of bread, because all restaurant bread is refined. Dip the vegetables in Balsamic vinaigrette.

---

[63] Jian-Wei Gu, et al., Ethanol stimulates tumor progression and expression of vascular endothelial growth factor in chick embryos, Cancer, Vol. 103, No. 2, 422-431. Researchers injected alcohol into chick embryos and the chicks had eight times more cancer cells in their blood vessels than chicks injected with saline. The researchers also noted significant increases in tumor size and tumor blood vessel density, as well as higher levels of the vascular endothelial growth factor, a protein involved in the growth of new blood vessels (that could feed tumors) in the alcohol-exposed embryos. Although these were large doses of alcohol, the researchers said that based on previous studies, that even light to moderate amounts of alcohol could induce new blood vessel growth for a tumor.

And during holiday gatherings with family and friends, eat before you get there to curb your appetite.

Following the RAVE Diet can be as simple or complicated as you want to make it. If you need recipes, look at the sample recipes in this book and explore the web site recipe links that contain thousands of delicious recipes (See *Recipes On The Web*) – but leave out any refined foods, animal foods and use vegetable oil substitutes. (See *Rules for Meal Preparation – Cooking Without Oil*)

For convenience, use frozen fruits and vegetables. They're almost as good as fresh and may be better in some cases due to modern storage and transportation techniques.

Coffee and many other stimulants - as well as alcohol - dehydrate your body and take more fluid out of it than they bring in. This contributes to cell dehydration, which some experts cite as the cause of premature aging. Avoid these products and make water your beverage of choice – it's the single best thing you can do for dry skin and wrinkles. By the way, dehydration and high blood sugar levels cause hangovers. The best way to prevent a hangover is to drink water before you go to bed. And take a walk the next morning to help burn off the excess sugar in your blood.

I'm sure most of you are thinking, yes, this all sounds good, but if I eat according to this pyramid, what a sacrifice! Actually, it's just the opposite. This diet is very indulgent because there are no restrictions on portion sizes.

Many people will agree with the health aspects of the RAVE Diet, but simply can't change their eating habits. First of all, everyone already eats plant foods. Rice, potatoes, lettuce, tomatoes, fruits, bread and so forth are all part of our diets and we all eat a wider range of plant foods than we realize, just too little of them. All you have to do is substitute that slice of steak or chicken on your plate – with *more* plant foods. You'll feel full and just as satisfied as you would with your standard American diet. Many studies have shown that potatoes are just as satisfying as meat – to meat-eaters – and there are hundreds of ways to prepare potatoes.

If you think you "hate" all vegetables, start by simply eating more of the familiar plant foods you do like – such as potatoes and brown rice. There are so many ways to "disguise" the taste of vegetables with seasonings and sauces that this shouldn't be a barrier. (See *Rules for Meal Preparation – Flavorings*.) You just have to get a little creative with your food preparation. This may be a challenge at first, but read up on how to prepare vegetables in this book and also what they can do for your body, which may make them go down a little easier.

Just as your taste for meat and dairy products was acquired, you can acquire a taste for foods you thought would be impossible to eat. Take bread, for example. If you buy good-tasting whole grain bread in the first place, you should enjoy the taste of the bread by itself, without any high-fat toppings. Try it. You can acquire the clean taste of "plain" bread after just a slice or two and you'll love it. Some people "hate" the taste of Portobello mushrooms. Trying grilling them with barbeque sauce or A1 steak sauce. They're delicious and a great substitute for hamburgers. And if you absolutely can't stand mushrooms (or another plant food), put them in food processor, then mix them into a meal.

Your tastes for food will change with this diet and you'll find you prefer the "cleaner" taste of natural foods. After eating this way, you'll find that high-fat foods will taste heavy and greasy and you'll notice that when you do eat high-fat foods, your entire system slows down and you feel sluggish.

Plant foods are bulky, which means you end up eating more food, in terms of quantity, but you'll actually consume fewer calories. One of the biggest problems is convenience in that you usually won't find healthy food at your local convenience store. This diet does not have to be inconvenient, you just have to think ahead and think in terms of whole plant foods. It's easy, once you get used to it. See *RAVE Diet Guidelines - Fast Food: Meals in Minutes* for a few suggestions along these lines.

Accelerating Weight Loss

If you want to accelerate your weight loss, follow these rules:

1) Eat only low-fat, plant foods that come in their natural packages.
2) Never skip meals, especially breakfast.
3) Drink at least a full glass of water half an hour before you eat to curb your appetite.
4) Eliminate breads, alcohol and salt.
5) Go light on all grain products and high-fat fruits and vegetables.
6) Go very light on nuts and nut products.
7) Make *low-fat vegetables the center of your diet.*
8) Snack on fruits because they contain water and fiber and are filling.
9) Try to eat at least one full meal salad a day with minimal dressing (make sure the dressing does not contain oil). In fact, a salad a day will not only keep the doctor away, but those pounds, as well.
10) Exercise before meals.
11) Follow the *No Exceptions* rule to the letter.

There is a time lag between the time you eat and the time you feel full. On a typical American diet, you could quickly gulp down 2,500 calories at one sitting – more than enough for a full day – and still not feel full. By taking time to eat, you give your stomach an opportunity to tell your brain that you're full. If you only have 5 – 10 minutes to eat a meal, don't try to feel full by eating more because you'll consume too many calories. You'll feel full in another 15 or 20 minutes. In the meantime, drink water and give your stomach enough time to send its message to your brain.

Also, get as much exercise as you can. Exercise not only does miraculous things for your health, but it will burn off those extra calories and tip your scales in the right direction. Exercise also curbs the appetite, so exercising before meals is the best time in terms of weight loss. There's no better way to lose weight than exercise and healthful eating.

One lady told me she was always hungry eating this diet. Her problem was that she was trying to lose weight the traditional way – by starving herself. She mistakenly felt that if she ate too much food she would gain weight. Eating the RAVE Diet is counter-intuitive because you should always eat when you're hungry. In the beginning, many people find they're eating more food than they ever ate in their lives, yet still losing weight. Don't be afraid to eat natural plant foods because they are very low in calories and fat. As your body adjusts to this new way of eating, you'll find your appetite will adjust, too. Just stick to it!

Another lady told me she wasn't losing weight. Her problem was that she was making too many exceptions and loading up on refined foods. If you make exceptions like this – and can't help it – then the only option you have is exercise. There's no magic bullet that will automatically reverse a sedentary lifestyle. Only you can do it by making exercise a daily part of your life.

Believe it or not, the *biggest* complaints I've had were from individuals who were afraid they were losing too much weight! When you get down near your ideal weight, your weight loss will stabilize and your appearance will be transformed. People may call you "skinny" only because we're used to seeing fat people as the norm. If you want to see someone at his ideal weight, take a look at Kevin Costner in the film "No Way Out." He looks terrific and that's how you can look, too, no matter what your age.

Visualizing Your Weight Loss Goal

There is a very simple, yet powerful, trick you can employ that will keep you on the RAVE Diet and enable you to resist temptation. What you should do is close your eyes and visualize what you will look like when you achieve your weight loss goal. Picture yourself running and playing, picture what you will look like in your new clothes, at social occasions and in every different situation you can imagine in your new lifestyle. In addition, visualize everything that you *associate* with your new lifestyle – a new attitude, confidence, new friends and so forth. No doubt, it is a very happy sight.

Spend a few minutes running these visualizations through your mind, then lock in the images. Do this frequently. You simply can't do it too often.

Every time you feel a craving for a food that is off the RAVE Diet, take a deep breath, close your eyes and run those images through your mind.

At the same time, imagine you have to make a journey in order to reach your new lifestyle. You have to walk a long way in order to get to your destination. Picture the food you want to eat as representing an obstacle to reaching your new lifestyle. Picture that food as a river you have to swim, a mountain you have to climb – or simply the most difficult obstacle you can imagine. That food you crave so deeply – that piece of chocolate or cheese – represents a setback that will keep you from reaching the lifestyle you want so badly. Each bite is going to set you back in your journey and make reaching your goal all the more difficult.

Some people make "vision boards" where they cut out pictures from magazines and newspapers and paste them onto a board. It ends up as a collage of images representing what their lifestyle goals are. After they have finished their collage, they hang it up in a place so they will see it every single day to remind them of what they are striving for.

There are an infinite number of variations to this theme. It's simply asserting mind over body in order to get you where you want your body to be. Always keep the positive images in your head. They will steer you in the right direction and keep you moving forward toward your new weight goal and lifestyle.

The RAVE Diet For Kids

The RAVE Diet is excellent for children. The questions and answers parents may have are much too extensive to be covered here and deserve special treatment, so a few references are provided below.

If you are an expectant mother, breast-feeding is probably the most important single thing you can do for your child. When we are born, our immune systems are weak. Mother's milk gives us the very first boost to our immune system.

Do not feed your child formulas. Breast fed babies are far healthier than formula-fed babies and *only mother's milk has immune strengthening nutrients*. And never, ever feed your child milk from any animal. Mother's milk is species-specific. Nature simply did not design animal milk for humans. Cow's milk is designed for baby calves, not humans. The only milk humans are designed to drink is human mother's milk – and then only as a baby.

Here are a few references that will answer your questions.

Books
Healthy Eating For Life For Children, Physicians Committee for Responsible Medicine
Raising Vegetarian Children, Joanne Stepaniak, Vesanto Melina
Disease-Proof Your Child, Joel Fuhrman, M.D.
Dr. Spock's Baby and Child Care, 7th Edition, Dr. Benjamin Spock

Web Sites
Vegetarian Baby and Child
      http://www.vegetarianbaby.com/
Articles on Vegetarian Parenting
      http://www.vegsource.com/parent/
Veg Family
      http://www.vegfamily.com/

What To Expect

I spent the last week eating no snacky stuff. I packed two lunches with me to work each day. When I got hungry in the afternoon, I reheated the second lunch and ate that. And I lost 2 pounds! I am really surprised that I can feel full and eat so much food and still lose weight. It's a strange feeling. I really didn't try cutting back on portions or doing anything "diety." My goal was simply to get through each afternoon without eating junk food. So I just took each day one at a time and ate rice, beans, vegetables, and fruits and ate enough to feel full. Thank you for your support and amazing film. Talk about life-changing. Best to you always, Chris (letter to the author)

Everyone is different and people will react somewhat differently to any new diet they adopt. You'll find you are eating far more food than you ever have in your life – and still losing weight. This is very different from typical dieting plans where you have to restrict portions in order to reduce caloric intake.
Here are just some of the possible changes you might experience when adopting the RAVE Diet.

Baseline Measurements: Eating habits can vary considerably even within the RAVE Diet guidelines, which is one of its strengths in that it can accommodate specialized diets within its overall boundaries. If you have trouble meeting the Baseline Measurement goals, e.g., your triglycerides are too high, always increase your consumption of low-fat vegetables and decrease your consumption of starchy vegetables, fruits and whole grains. In other words, aim toward the middle of the RAVE Diet food pyramid and make *low-fat vegetables* the center of your diet. In short, go for the greens – particularly leafy green vegetables – and cut back on the grains. Try that for a month and your results will improve dramatically.

Cravings: Some people experience cravings for some foods, particularly sweets, chocolate and cheese.[64] Hard as this may be to believe, these are withdrawal symptoms that are not totally uncommon when switching to the RAVE Diet. Such foods are actually addictive and food manufacturers have invested heavily in juggling ingredients to make foods as addictive as possible. The problem is that we've lost our taste for real food because most food we eat today is smothered with salt, fat, sweets and chemicals. As a result, your taste buds are currently "warped." It normally takes about three weeks for tastes to change. If you stick with the RAVE Diet, your cravings for the "highs" of sugar, fat and salt will go away as your taste buds return to normal boundaries. If you don't think you can resist these cravings, think of transition foods, such as soy ice cream instead of regular ice cream. (See *RAVE Diet Guidelines - Transition Foods*.) And remember to use the visualization techniques described above to resist temptation. (See *The RAVE Diet & Lifestyle - Visualizing Your Weight Loss Goal*.)

Hunger In-Between Meals: Some people get hungry before lunch, others in mid-afternoon, depending on the meal beforehand. This happens most often with people who are trying to lose weight because they will cut back on portions. This is a mistake on the RAVE Diet because all the foods are low calorie to begin with. Some people will eat only fruit for breakfast and get hungry before noon. Add whole grain products to your breakfast, such as oatmeal, and whole wheat bread. (By the way, oatmeal is *the* most filling breakfast food.) If you eat salads for lunch, make it a meal salad (think big!) and add a handful of beans. Or have a baked potato with it or another side dish. If you're at work, bring your own food and make sure you have enough to snack on if you need to. (See *RAVE Diet Guidelines – Fast Food: Meals In Minutes*.) At dinner, use brown rice or potatoes to fill you up. Don't be afraid to eat because you'll probably consume a larger quantity of food on the RAVE Diet than you did previously – until your body adjusts. The quantity is not as important as the type of foods you're eating. Remember, this is a long-term diet and it's much better to lose the pounds slowly and comfortably because you're establishing new eating habits for the rest of your life. The hunger in-between meals is usually the result of consuming fewer calories – which is, after all, the point of this diet. Your body has to adjust to the caloric decline slowly, so *increase* the portion size at first so you don't get hungry later.

Constipation Cured: A good bowel movement is one of the most under-appreciated aspects of American life. With the RAVE Diet, your constipation will be cured and, for most, this will be the biggest immediate change. You'll not

---

[64] Many find cheese and chocolate to be the most difficult foods to give up. Part of the reason for this has to do with the casomorphin in cow's milk, which has a subtle addicting and pain-killing quality about it. So yes, Marge, there is morphine in cow's milk. Ever wonder where that chocolate "high" came from?

only experience bowel movements like you've never had them before, but you'll also be getting rid of toxic substances in your body on a regular basis. And if you're accustomed to reading the newspaper while sitting on the toilet, that pastime will be history because you won't have time! Nor will you experience the straining you used to put up with (which can result in varicose veins). Some people will find they have two to three bowel movements a day (one after every meal). Far from being abnormal, this is actually the ideal. Parenthetically, constipation (and the accompanying straining) is a common side effect of "low-carb" diets. It's not surprising that profits of laxative makers skyrocket when low-carb diets are the craze.[65] Our intent is to put these businesses out of business because once you've adopted the RAVE Diet, you'll never have to take a laxative again.

Detoxification: What you will be doing on this diet is a natural form of detoxification. Most of us have a lot of toxicity stored within our cellular tissue. As soon as the shift is made to more natural foods, the body will begin to release toxins. The high fiber content of the diet will bind with toxins in your system (e.g., mercury) and take them out of your system the same way fiber binds with cholesterol, excess sex hormones and other substances and removes them. At first, a very small percentage of individuals may feel a lack of energy or fatigue, as well as other side effects of eating healthy. This is the result of the body detoxifying itself. People who quit smoking often experience exactly the same feelings. Stick with it! This will pass as your body gets rid of toxins and adjusts to this new way of eating. Your energy will return and return at a much higher level than before. Other people have experienced headaches. This is similar to withdrawal from caffeine. Again, stick with it. This is a classic sign of detoxification and the headaches or other side effects will go away.

Initial Gas: Due to the high fiber content of the RAVE Diet, you may experience more flatulence than normal. As your body transitions to the RAVE Diet, however, that problem will go away and you won't have any more gas than you did on your old diet. A side benefit: The gas from eating plant foods is nowhere near as smelly as the gas you get from eating animal foods (scientific fact). You'll also find that not only your breath, but also your body odor is much sweeter smelling. Parenthetically, refined plant products, such as refined soy products cause more gas than whole, natural plant foods.

Not Eating Animal Food: Some will, no doubt, experience anxiety because they think they're going to miss out on an essential nutrient by not eating animal foods. (See *Notes – Protein*.) This is a measure of the brainwashing we have all experienced, not only from the meat and dairy industries, but also from our own government, doctors and dieticians. Trust me, only good health will result. This is, after all, the way humans have been eating throughout our history. A neighbor of mine told me that he couldn't sleep without having a slab of steak or chicken

---

[65] AP, "Diet Trends May Broaden Demographics," 3/30/04.

before he went to bed. He was clinically obese and still is. *You* won't have any problems sleeping on this diet. In fact, I wish I had a dime for everyone who told me how good he or she felt by *not* eating animals. You will, too, and it just may help you sleep more soundly.

Pleasure Traps: We're living in a sea of food advertisements which constantly tell us it's "Ok" to eat bad foods. During holidays, in particular, your friends will encourage you to eat bad foods and it's difficult to resist these temptations. This is the "Pleasure Trap," and often results in backsliding and getting away from the RAVE Diet altogether. Once you do that, the weight will return and you'll be back where you started. Simply stated, the Pleasure Trap means you will be caught in a trap of immediate pleasure, which undermines the long-term goals you have set for yourself. You'll be sacrificing long-term pleasures (being slim and the lifestyle that goes with that) for the short-term pleasures of high sugar, salt and fatty foods. What to do if you fall off the wagon? The first thing I'd suggest is that you get some blood work done to see how out of whack your measurements are against the *Baseline Measurements* spelled out in this book. That should provide some incentive to get off the animal or refined foods. If you find yourself caught in the Pleasure Trap, here is what I would suggest: Get off the animal and refined foods completely for at least three weeks. The process of withdrawal is not all that different from what one experiences with cigarettes. It takes about three weeks to change your taste buds – roughly the same amount of time it takes a smoker to really feel he or she is over the nicotine hump. And just as cigarettes will always be a lure to a smoker, so too will animal and refined foods to someone who was once addicted to them. Stay away from these foods for at least three weeks and the cravings should come under control, if they're not gone altogether. Find substitutes in herbs, spices and sauces. As your taste buds get used to these flavors, you will come to prefer them. Get smart and follow the RAVE admonition "No Exceptions" – and stick with it. The long-term rewards are far too great to sacrifice for short-term pleasures that will only wind up on your belly and butt.

Carbophobia Conquered: You'll be able to enjoy carbohydrates of all varieties – so long as they are made from *whole,* natural foods. The carbohydrates you should rightly be afraid of are from refined foods. One misconception about high carbohydrate diets is that they raise triglycerides (blood fats). This is a common misconception based on tests done with *refined* or simple carbohydrates, which will raise triglycerides. If you're eating only *complex* carbs found in natural foods, triglyceride levels will not go up. In fact, the best way to dramatically reduce triglycerides is to follow the RAVE Diet because the combination of complex carbohydrates and exercise will reduce triglycerides better than any other approach. (In a few people, who are sensitive, any form of fruit will raise triglycerides because the primary sugar is fructose, a simple sugar.) There is so much confusion about carbohydrates, it would take a book to sort them out. Instead, just remember the refined carbohydrates are the bad guys, while whole-food carbs are the good guys.

Sniping Remarks From Uninformed "Friends": In social occasions, I normally do not bring up diet, but if you are eating, it's often inevitable. A remark often heard by people is that low-fat diets are dangerous. This is how strange our attitudes toward food are. The fact we consider a diet that actually reverses diseases to be dangerous is nothing short of outrageous! Yet the diet your friends are on – which causes diseases – is considered safe! People who call low-fat diets dangerous are, in fact, eating the most dangerous diet in the world. People eating RAVE-like diets are in excellent health throughout the world and are not killed off with cardiovascular disease, our common cancers, diabetes and our other major diseases. A low-fat diet is the healthiest – and safest – diet in the world. Billions can attest to that. Unfortunately, very few are Americans and I'm sure very few are your friends.

Better Skin: Because you are clearing out your blood vessels, the blood flow carrying oxygen and nutrients throughout your body will be greatly enhanced and will produce some amazing results. Some people have even had "liver" or "sun spots" disappear from their skin when they adopted this diet. Other people have told me that if they don't consume oils, their skin will dry out. This is a misconception, and a greasy one. Most people have dry skin because they are dehydrated due to their diet. Restrict your consumption of diuretics, which take more fluid out of your body than they bring in – and increase your consumption of plain water and plant foods (which contain high amounts of water). Doing this will keep your skin moist and fresh and do more for your wrinkles than any skin cream on the market. The most common diuretics are coffee, tea and similar stimulants, as well as alcohol.

Better Senses: Largely as a result of opening up your blood vessels, there will be a range of changes you will notice over time, including better hearing, eyesight, taste, smell and touch.

Cheaper Grocery Bill: Many complain about the higher cost of organic foods, but overall, you will save money on groceries. One estimate, made some years ago, pegged the savings at around $1,400 a year. If fruits and vegetables are expensive in your area, use frozen fruits and vegetables instead of fresh. Frozen produce is often packed at the peak of freshness and will also taste better than out-of-season produce. The big savings with the RAVE Diet is not on groceries, however, but current and future health care and medication costs.

Blaming the Diet? Don't blame this diet for coincidental things that may happen to you either physically or mentally. I've heard everything from a man's hair turning gray, to someone's depression blamed on this diet. Don't worry. Your nails, hair and everything else will continue to grow just fine, if not better than ever. The only thing you may experience are anxiety attacks because you think you're not getting enough protein or calcium, especially after you watch the next food advertisement on television. You'll get over it. A year after adopting this diet, you'll have a completely different view of food that will make your doctor smile at your next checkup.

Food Sensitivities/Allergies: In rare cases, the increase in consumption of whole plant foods may trigger food sensitivities or food allergies with certain foods simply because you are eating more of them. In these cases, it is a matter of finding out which foods are triggers and eliminating them from your diet or cutting back on them. For specific information on a variety of "trigger" foods, get a copy of *Foods That Fight Pain, Neal Barnard, M.D.* A few have experienced gluten intolerance, or Celiac Disease. This is the result of eating more wheat-related foods. The RAVE Diet did not cause the Celiac Disease. You always had an intolerance for gluten (the protein in wheat-related foods) and the diet just brought it out due to increased consumption of wheat. There is a simple solution. Stop eating all forms of wheat (including durum, semolina, spelt, kamut, einkorn and faro) and related grains such as rye, barley and triticale. You can substitute rice, potatoes, etc. or there are gluten-free products that are becoming increasingly available.

If you are already in good health, the changes will be subtle and you will find you will be in even better health over the long-term. If you have an eating-related disease, such as heart disease, the changes can be dramatic, such as those described by Dr. Neal Pinckney in the film *Eating*. Dr. Pinckney was scheduled for an emergency bypass operation. He walked away from the operation, changed to the RAVE Diet and within just two weeks, he cleared up his severe angina. After just seven months, his heart disease had been reversed and he completed an eight-mile marathon run. He accomplished this by simply changing the way he ate. No bypass, no stents, no drugs, no nothing!

If you have any one of a myriad of eating-related diseases, these can be treated and cured with diet. Check our web site (www.RaveDiet.com) for a list of health providers who treat diseases naturally using diet.

Sex, Booze, Rock 'n Roll

"I wouldn't recommend sex, drugs or insanity for everyone, but they've always worked for me." – Hunter S. Thompson

The Sex Diet

Now that I have your attention, let me explain that the Sex Diet is very simple and easy to follow. Instead of having a meal, you simply have sex. Anyone who's tried this will tell you it's a great way to lose weight. It not only reduces caloric intake, but burns off those extra calories, as well. Naturally, I tried this for a while and must say I had a great time and lost weight, but unfortunately, it can't go on forever. There are, however, many ways in which the RAVE Diet can make your sex life explosive without your ever skipping a single meal.

The two key aspects of the RAVE Diet that will revitalize your sex life are: 1) by opening up your arteries – yes the ones supplying blood to your genital area (this goes for both male and female) – and 2) with exercise.

By eliminating animal products and refined foods, you won't become impotent due to damage caused to the arteries supplying blood to the penis.[66] Men with high cholesterol levels are more likely to experience erectile dysfunction[67] and the high levels of environmental chemicals concentrated in meat wreak havoc on testosterone levels, resulting in decreased ejaculate volume, lower sperm counts, poor sperm motility and infertility.[68]

It's ironic that Viagra was originally developed to treat the pain caused by angina, a condition brought on by the same cause as impotence – a high-fat and cholesterol-laden diet. Viagra, of course, did not help angina, but test subjects found – much to their delight – it solved another problem they were experiencing as a result of their diets.

The second element of the RAVE Diet – exercise – will add years to your sex life, improve your self-image, mental clarity, reduce stress, rev up your sex drive – no matter what your age – and will result in better erections.[69]

By opening up your arteries and getting plenty of exercise, you'll find your sex life rising like a Phoenix from the ashes, so to speak. And once that happens, there are hosts of benefits from having frequent sex. Here are just a few:

- Improved sense of smell (production of the hormone prolactin surges)
- Reduced risk of heart disease (sex reduces risk of heart attack or stroke)
- Weight loss (hey, if nothing else, it's exercise)
- Reduced depression (who wouldn't be happy after sex?)
- Boosts the immune system (you feel invincible!)
- Pain relief (levels of the hormone oxytocin surge)
- Less frequent colds and flu (strengthens the immune system)
- Better bladder control (similar to Kegel exercises)

---

[66] Feldman HA. Erectile dysfunction and coronary risk factors: prospective results from the Massachusetts male aging study. Prev. Med. 2000 Apr;30(4):328-38.

[67] Bodie J. Laboratory evaluations of erectile dysfunction: an evidence based approach. J Urol. 2003 Jun;169(6):2262-4.

[68] Rozati R . Role of environmental estrogens in the deterioration of male factor fertility. Fertil Steril. 2002 Dec;78(6):1187-94.

[69] Sexual Function in Men Older Than 50 Years of Age: Results from the Health Professionals Follow-up Study, Constance G. Bacon, ScD; Murray A. Mittleman, MD, ScD; Ichiro Kawachi, MD, PhD; Edward Giovannucci, MD, ScD; Dale B. Glasser, PhD; and Eric B. Rimm, ScD, Vol. 139, Issue 3, 161-68.

- Better teeth (seminal plasma contains minerals shown to reduce tooth decay...)
- A happier prostate (lower chance of prostate cancer with more sex[70])

Insofar as booze is concerned, one of the best things you can do to lose weight is to cut it out because alcohol is nothing but empty calories. Okay, okay. I know it does other things for you besides pack on the pounds. But if you're going to drink, avoid mixed drinks and drink only *before* you have sex.

If you're looking for a truly out-of-this-world sexual experience, there is one absolute best time to drink: *after* you exercise and *before* you have sex, because both will get you in the mood. (Trust me, I've done a little study on this.) The combination of exercise and a little booze will do wonders for your sex life, so get exercising, have a drink, jump into bed and live a little!

And insofar as rock 'n roll goes, well, in this context, no further comment is necessary...

The Pursuit of Happiness

"There are people who have money, and there are people who are rich."
– Coco Chanel

"The goal in life is to die young – as late as possible." – Ashley Montagu

The relationship between diet and disease is as old as the Bible. You may recall the biblical story of Daniel. After suffering through ill health, Daniel made a radical proposal to take the servants off their rich, royal diet and put them on a diet of vegetables and water. In only ten days, the servants looked healthier and better nourished than any of the other men who had eaten the rich, royal foods.

You don't have to eat just vegetables and water to achieve the health of Daniel's servants and the remainder of this book shows you how to eat a wide variety of delicious foods that will do wonders for your health and well-being.

The RAVE Diet is an elegantly simple solution to the health problems that are tearing apart the very fabric of our lives. Instead of complicated drugs and surgery, diet can replace them all and bring simplicity to your health and balance to your life.

Our bodies are incredibly smart. We have *trillions* of cells intricately and automatically coordinating their activities so we can go on with our lives without having to worry about our health. But when we introduce bad foods to our bodies, we start to destroy this finely tuned masterpiece, balance is lost and the

---

[70] Michael F. Leitzmann; et al. Ejaculation Frequency and Subsequent Risk of Prostate Cancer. JAMA. 2004;291:1578-1586.

preconditions for disease set in. Our bodies scramble to recover and regain balance, but so long as bad food keeps coming in, they will remain out of balance and, over time, disease will take over. Our bodies are extremely forgiving of bad habits – but only up to a point – and when they have had enough, people will get a wakeup call like they've never had before.

What most Americans – and medical experts – consider to be a balanced diet today is radically tipped toward heart disease, cancer, diabetes, obesity and all the other health problems we are now experiencing. One of the favorite lines of doctors is that "…as we age, we tend to get…." But this is nonsense. Do you think a large belly is the result of aging? A big butt? Do you think osteoporosis automatically comes with age? Arthritis? Heart disease? Our common cancers? We get these diseases as we age because of a lifetime of bad eating habits, coupled with a sedentary lifestyle.

Those people who want to improve their health, but will not change their diets, are in for bad times down the road. It's like people who want a well-financed retirement, but won't save money. They will end up with a very difficult retirement. And so will those who don't start investing in themselves by changing their diet.

How many days do you have in your life? If you live to 75, you have about 27,000 days of living on this earth. I used to think 27,000 days was a lot. I also used to think $27,000 was a lot – until I was nearly out of money. Then those last few precious dollars seemed like a fortune. It works the same way with life.

Remember how long it was between the time you were 10 and 20? Imagine adding the same number of high quality years to the end of your life by just changing your eating habits and getting a modest amount of exercise.

The RAVE Diet is not about adding years to your life so much as it's about raising the *quality* of your life by avoiding diseases and drugs[71] and making the last third of your life just as vigorous as the first third.

For me, the measure of a good life is how much happiness you get out of it. To me, the pursuit of happiness is really about owning *less* stuff, while gaining *more* purpose in life. "Stuff" brings temporary pleasure. Purpose brings lasting pleasure. People who look outside of themselves for happiness by pursuing "stuff" are always disappointed because long-term happiness inevitably springs from within. The same can be said for your health. Health *always* comes before wealth and you must remind yourself of that when setting your priorities.

---

[71] The typical person 65 years or older takes a dozen or more medications a day. Only the first one or two drugs are actually prescribed to deal with the original medical problem. The others are required to deal with the side effects of the original two, plus the interactions of all the other drugs they are taking. There are more than 2 million drug reactions in the US annually and more than 100,000 reactions are fatal. And due to recording anomalies, it's been estimated the figure should be much higher, like 700,000 deaths a year. Sadly, in over 95 percent of all cases, the original problem for which the medical was prescribed could have been resolved naturally.

Depression is the consequence of seeking excessive stimulation. When you strive to experience extreme "highs," you will inevitably end up depressed when the exhilaration from those highs wears off. Always seek to find your middle ground. Balance your life. Seek purpose in it and go for more than just the temporary, immediate highs life has to offer.

For every immediate pleasure you give up, you gain something more valuable and lasting. The smoker or alcoholic who gives up his destructive habit gains much more than he loses. You will gain much more by giving up the "pleasure traps" of animal and refined foods – without exception. I've seen people transformed by the RAVE Diet. I've seen men, who used to grill steaks on the barbeque during football games, now talking about the best way to make chopped salad. You'll feel good about yourself and what you're doing – not only for your own health, but also for the world we all live in.

Dare to be different. Change your life and seek long-term happiness from within by adopting a lifestyle that I guarantee will pay countless dividends throughout your entire life.

Notes

Protein

When you ask the typical American, "Where does protein come from?" they'll stammer for a moment and then say something like, "From meat, dairy and eggs." And they'll be dead wrong. Protein doesn't come from any of these sources. All protein on the planet comes from plants. In fact, protein is the result of the interaction of sunlight on plants. Although many people don't think plants have protein at all, plants are the mothers of *all* the protein we eat.

Most people think only animal products have protein, but the lawn in your front yard is full of protein. You may not recognize it, but a cow would. Herbivores, such as cows, eat plants to get their protein. When carnivores eat herbivores, they are actually eating the protein that originally came from the plants eaten by herbivores. The problem with eating protein from animals is that it comes in a package of saturated fat and cholesterol, the two most deadly ingredients in the American diet.

For most Americans, getting enough protein simply means eating animal foods. You'll have doctors and dieticians flatly state that you won't get enough protein by just eating plant foods. Unfortunately, they are following the protein requirements of our government, which have been set by the meat, dairy and egg industries through lobbying efforts – and they are not only ridiculously high, but also potentially dangerous. Because this standard has the flag wrapped around it, nutritionists and health professionals have taken it as "science" and preach this gospel to the public. They are, in fact, mindlessly acting as sales persons for industries selling high-protein foods, which have paid off politicians.

A friend recently went to her nutritionist who said that in order to get the protein her body requires purely from vegetables, she would need to consume more vegetables than she could possibly eat. This is not only scientifically false, but an affront to common sense because if that were true, the human race would not have made it to the 20th century.

It's extremely easy to meet protein needs on virtually any diet. In fact, you'd have to be starving not to get enough protein eating anything other than a junk food diet.

Here's a simple quiz for you. Which has more protein? Steak, broccoli or spinach? Spinach has the most protein, then broccoli and steak comes in last place.

The USDA dietary guidelines call for protein levels above 10 percent of total calories. Ten percent is four times what the average adult actually needs (see below). This exaggeration, unfortunately, is not based on human needs, but the needs of food lobbies selling high-protein foods.

The protein in human mother's milk is only five percent of total calories. Mother's milk is providing protein during the fastest growth period humans will ever experience outside the womb. At no other time in our lives will we need a greater amount of protein. In fact, the average adult needs only half that amount, or two and one-half percent of calories from protein.[1]

Since 1974, the World Health Organization (WHO) has recognized this, but they doubled their recommendation to 5 percent of total calories in order to account for infants and people who are sick. Guess what? The WHO recommendation is exactly what mother's milk provides.

Now, why would the U.S. Government – or anyone else for that matter – recommend anything greater than five percent? Unfortunately, any protein standard higher than five percent is due to money and lobbying, not science.

Most of us would say, well, there's no harm in getting too much protein. But, in fact, there is potentially great harm because high protein diets can result in kidney disease, osteoporosis, cardiovascular disease and cancers.

If you're eating more protein than your body needs to repair tissue, it's burned as a fuel. Unfortunately, protein is both an inefficient fuel and a dirty fuel. It's inefficient because you have to expend more energy to take protein molecules apart than you do to break down carbohydrates and fats, due to the complicated structure of protein. It's dirty because protein contains nitrogen. Instead of producing clean carbon dioxide and water, burning protein produces nitrogenous residues that not only are irritating to the immune system and toxic to the liver, but also put a big workload on the kidneys. High-protein diets can also cause fatigue, digestive strain and aggravation of allergies and autoimmune diseases.

Given all this, why are our protein requirements so high? There is some dubious "science" behind the political efforts of food industries to raise our protein requirements. This science hinges on studies involving rats. In fact, the USDA protein requirements for Americans are based on the nutritional needs of *rats*. The very first study was done back in 1914, but subsequent studies with rats have continued since then and have formed the basis, i.e., the "science," behind our protein requirements. Needless to say, the high-protein food industries embraced these studies as if they were manna from heaven.

In the excitement over these studies, it apparently never occurred to anyone that rats are highly inappropriate for the study of human protein requirements. Rats do not eat like humans, digest food like humans, metabolize food like humans, grow like humans and their protein requirements are not at all like humans. In addition, mother's milk from rats is a whopping 49 percent of calories (vs. five percent for human mother's milk), and the amino acid profiles for rats are not at all like human amino acid profiles. This shouldn't come as a

---

[1] Minimum protein requirements of adults, Hegsted, D., Am. J. Clin. Nutr. 21: 3520; The amino acid requirements of man. XIII The sparing effect of cystine on methionine requirement, Rose, W.C. and Wixom, R.L., J. Biol. Chem., 216, 763-773.

big surprise to most of you because, among other things, just comparing a rat and a human should tell you right off there are monumental differences between the two species. But this incidental fact did not deter the "scientists" from their work and making our protein requirements "rat-like" to this day.

In every study conducted with humans, protein from plant foods exceeded human nutritional requirements. Studies in which humans were fed wheat bread alone - or potatoes alone - or corn alone - or rice alone - have all shown that humans were able to meet their protein needs and get all the essential amino acids they needed.[2] And vegetables have an average protein content of 25 percent of calories, far in excess of what we need.[3]

But the rat standard for protein has led us into even more difficulties because people have embraced the notion of a "complete" protein and pointed to eggs as the gold standard. This gold standard, however, is based on the nutritional needs of *rats*. In fact, the human body does quite well on foods containing "incomplete" proteins because the body is smart enough to mix and match amino acids in order to form a complete protein and meet the body's needs. In fact, the first thing the body does when it encounters a "complete" protein is break it apart into an incomplete protein, so it can mix and match amino acids according to the body's current needs. The whole notion of a "complete" protein is outdated, based on worthless "science," and should be discarded because it does not apply to human beings. Nor does the current U.S. government standard for protein.

Vitamin D

If there is a single micronutrient that practically all Americans are deficient in, it is vitamin D, known as the "sunshine" vitamin – and having adequate amount of this vitamin is critical in fighting a wide variety of diseases, especially cancer.[4]

---

[2] Kofranyi, E., Jekat, F. and Muller-Wecker, H. (1970). 'The minimum protein requirements of humans, tested with mixtures of whole egg plus potatoes and maize plus beans', Z. Physiol. Chem., 351, 1485-1493; Clark, H.E., Malzer, J.L., Onderka, H.M., Howe, J.M. and Moon, W. (1973). 'Nitrogen balances of adult human subjects fed combinations of wheat, beans, corn, milk, and rice', Am. J. Clin. Nutr., 26, 702-706; Edwards, C.H., Booker, L.K., Rumph, C.H., Wright, W.G. and Ganapathy, S.N. (1971). 'Utilisation of wheat by adult man; nitrogen metabolism, plasma amino acids and lipids', Am. J. Clin. Nutr., 24, 181-193; Lee, C., Howe, J.M., Carlson, K. and Clark, H.E. (1971). 'Nitrogen retention of young men fed rice with or without supplementary chicken', Am. J. Clin. Nutr., 24, 318-323; Kies, C., Williams, E. and Fox, H.M. (1965). 'Determination of first limiting nitrogenous factor in corn protein for nitrogen retention in human adults', J. Nutr., 86, 350-356.

[3] Eat To Live, Joel Fuhrman, M.D., p. 52.

[4] Grant WB. An estimate of premature cancer mortality in the U.S. due to inadequate doses of solar ultraviolet-B radiation. Cancer 2002;94:1867-75; Hanchette CL and

Vitamin D is also important for bones as it facilitates the absorption of calcium into the bone and a vitamin D deficiency will allow only a fraction of the calcium available to be absorbed by the bone.[5]

Because of our lifestyles, we simply do not get out in the sun much, which accounts for the deficiency. Of course, there are vitamin D supplements but, again, they cannot hold a candle to the "supercharged" vitamin D you can get naturally because it is much more powerful than the synthetic vitamin D available in supplements.[6]

Unfortunately, sunscreens block the production of vitamin D, so you have to get a little sunlight *before* you put on sunscreen. Also, you should allow full-spectrum sunlight to enter your eyes, so avoid wearing sunglasses.

Here are some general rules of thumb: during the summer, from 10 a.m. to 2 p.m. (the angle of the sun is important), fair-skinned people should get just 10 minutes of exposure, while very dark-skinned people should get 30 minutes, several times a week. Those with skin colors in-between can adjust accordingly. You should expose about 25% of your body, i.e., face, hands and arms or arms and legs. Use your common sense and never, ever allow yourself to come close to being sunburned. In fact, if you know how long it will take before you burn, about one-quarter of that time would be adequate. Moderate sunlight exposure during the summer is enough to allow you to maintain healthy vitamin D levels throughout the year because the body stores this vitamin and releases it as needed.

If you cannot get out in the sun, especially in the winter months, the recommended supplement dosage should be about 1,000 IU a day.[7] The government has set the safe upper limit at 2,000 IU a day.[8]

Schwartz GG. Geographic patterns of prostate cancer mortality. Evidence for a protective effect of ultraviolet radiation. Cancer 1992;70:2861-9. Note that vitamin D has receptors in more than 36 organs throughout the body, which means a deficiency of this vitamin will affect a wide variety of health issues.

[5] Chapuy, M.C., Preziosi, P., Maaner, M., Arnaud, S., Galan, P., Hercberg, S., and Meunier, P.J. (1997). Prevalance of vitamin D insufficiency in an adult normal population. Osteoporosis International 7: 439-443. The classic illustration of our bones' need for vitamin D is rickets, a disease characterized by soft and deformed bones. Before vitamin D supplementation, the cure for rickets was simply to get children into sunlight so their bodies could make vitamin D. Floating Hospital in Boston originally got its name because it was a large boat that, in the summertime, took children with rickets into Boston Harbor to be bathed in sunshine in order to cure their disease.

[6] The China Study, T. Colin Campbell, p. 180; The UV Advantage, Michael F. Holick.

[7] Taken from The UV Advantage, Michael F. Holick, Ph.D., p. 150. Vitamin D recommendations vary widely. And as our knowledge increases about this vitamin, the recommended dosage goes up. See also, Wolpowitz D, Gilchrest BA., The vitamin D questions: how much do you need and how should you get it? J Am Acad Dermatol. 2006 Feb;54(2):301-17; Reichrath J, The challenge resulting from positive and negative effects of sunlight: how much solar UV exposure is appropriate to balance between

Despite the bad publicity regarding indoor tanning facilities, they can be safe if you do it responsibly and – most important – the facility uses low-pressure lamps, which emit a balance of UVA and UVB rays.

Because of the PR job done by institutions such as the American Cancer Society, many people are practically hysterical about exposing their skin to the sun for fear of getting skin cancer. This hysteria is not justified and can actually do severe damage to your health. In fact, the highest rates of melanoma, the most deadly skin cancer, are found in people who spend most of their time indoors away from the sun, and melanomas usually occur in parts of the body that receive no sun exposure. In addition, there is no credible scientific evidence that moderate sun exposure causes melanomas.[9] In fact, there are many scientific studies showing a lower incidence of melanoma when people are regularly exposed to sunlight.[10] People who received a lot of sun exposure up to the time of their melanoma diagnosis had better survival rates than those who received little sun exposure.[11]

Keep in mind that when we are sunburned, the redness is caused by blood rushing to the skin in order to repair damaged cells and destroy any that have turned cancerous. If your immune system is running on empty, the repair job will be less than perfect, leaving cancer cells behind to multiply – which goes a long way in explaining why we have a skin cancer epidemic in this country, despite spending less time outdoors than our forebears. With a strong immune system, there won't be a problem. And, in fact, squamous cell and basel cell cancers should easily go away with this diet.

The consumption of animal protein has a tendency to block the production of the vitamin D we receive from the sun, thereby reducing the amount of "supercharged" vitamin D available to our bodies.[12] This is just another reason to eliminate animal products from our diets. Bottom line? A good diet can do more

---

risks of vitamin D deficiency and skin cancer? Prog Biophys Mol Biol. 2006 Sep;92(1):9-16; Vieth R. What is the optimal vitamin D status for health? Prog Biophys Mol Biol. 2006 Sep;92(1):26-32.

[8] Taken from the Harvard Medical School Family Guide. See www.health.harvard.edu/fhg/updates/update0204a.shtml

[9] The UV Advantage, Michael F. Holick, Ph.D., p. 14.

[10] Berwick M, Armstrong BK, Ben-Porat L, et al., Sun exposure and mortality from melanoma. J Natl Cancer Inst. 2005;97:195-199; Millen AE, Tucker MA, Hartge P, et al., Diet and melanoma in a case-control study. Cancer Epidemiol Biomarkers Prev. 2004;13:1042-1051.

[11] Berwick M, Armstrong BK, Ben-Porat L, et al., Sun exposure and mortality from melanoma. J Natl Cancer Inst. 2005;97:195-199.

[12] The China Study, T. Colin Campbell, Ph.D., p. 180.

to thwart skin cancer than staying away from the sun. Sun exposure should be encouraged because the benefits for cancer prevention[13] are incalculable.

Problems with the Glycemic Index

One of the latest trends in nutrition is a simple-minded, single-variable analysis called the Glycemic Index (GI), which almost every major authority in the country has embraced, despite its serious flaws. Why have they embraced such a flawed tool? Because it has the air of "science" behind it – the GI categorizes foods by simple numbers. Hence, a food can be categorized by a number and placed on a scale. Unfortunately, the GI is of little practical value, despite the fact that there are a number of diets out there based solely on this dubious tool.

The Glycemic Index was designed to measure the effect of a *single food* on blood sugar levels. And that is a big problem. If we were to eat a single food for a meal, the GI might be of limited value. Unfortunately, few people eat a single food for a meal. Factors which throw off the GI in the real world are the mix of fiber, fat and protein in foods comprising a meal, how refined the ingredients are, whether the food was cooked, fried, how ripe a fruit is, etc.

Another problem is that the GI may predict the effect of a single food on blood sugar levels, but it does not accurately predict how much insulin the body will release in response to a rise in blood sugar – and *this is far more important than blood sugar levels*. As a result, the GI produces very strange results. Lentils, which are good according to the index, actually provoke *higher insulin levels* than potatoes, which are bad, according to the index. A fried potato, containing artery-clogging trans fats, is better than a baked potato. Adding vinegar to a meal can lower the GI of any food and – believe it or not – adding sugar to a food has *no effect* on the index. Ice cream, according to the index, is better for you than whole wheat bread. Sugar-sweetened chocolate is better for you than carrots and a Mars candy bar is better for you than a potato.

Advocates of high-protein diets, say that eating carbohydrates raises insulin levels and therefore causes weight gain, while eating animal proteins and fats does not. They are dead wrong. Beef raises insulin levels more than *refined,*

---

[13] Holick MF, Vitamin D: importance in the prevention of cancers, type 1 diabetes, heart disease, and osteoporosis. Am J Clin Nutr. 2004 Mar;79(3):362-71; Robsahm TE, Tretli S, Dahlback A, Moan J, Vitamin D3 from sunlight may improve the prognosis of breast-, colon- and prostate cancer (Norway), Cancer Causes Control. 2004 Mar;15(2):149-58; Zhou W, Suk R, et al., Vitamin D is associated with improved survival in early-stage non-small cell lung cancer patients, Cancer Epidemiol Biomarkers Prev. 2005 Oct;14(10):2303-9; Berwick M, Armstrong BK, et al., Sun exposure and mortality from melanoma, J Natl Cancer Inst. 2005 Feb 2;97(3):195-9.

white pasta and *27 times* more than brown rice. And fish raises insulin levels more than whole grain bread.[14]

In fact, most of the foods with low GI's are fruits, vegetables, grains, beans and whole grains, the very foods such low-carb diets say you should avoid.

This is just a small sampling of the incoherent contradictions involved with the Glycemic Index that not only defy common sense, but science. The GI is so unreliable that the American Diabetes Association does not recommend using the index in the prevention or treatment of diabetes. Because of all these contradictions, the GI is of little practical value in determining what you should be eating and boils down to little more than a red herring that some Diet Doctors are using to distract people from good nutrition.

Forget the Glycemic Index. There is a better, simpler and more reliable measure. Instead of focusing on numbers, choose whole, natural plant foods and you will always be eating the best foods you can buy.

Osteoporosis and Acidic Diets

"In fact, the scientific literature states clearly that a "calcium deficiency disease" due to a low calcium intake from natural diets simply does not exist. In other words, all diets provide adequate calcium to meet our health needs...." - John A. McDougall, McDougall's Medicine

Your entire body chemistry changes according to the type of food you eat and that has consequences to your health. Because of our change in diet during the last century, American bodies have become very acidic and virtually all degenerative diseases ranging from cancers to tooth decay – are associated with excess acidity in our bodies.

Blood acid levels are measured on a pH scale from 1 to 14. Ideally, your blood should be slightly alkaline at 7.4. A soda, for example, has a pH of 2 and is highly acidic, whereas tap water has a pH of 8.4, which is very alkaline.

There are three ways to make your blood less acidic: First, eat more plant foods because plant foods are alkaline and have a higher percentage of water than other foods. Second, drink more water. Not water containing anything else, just plain, simple water. Third, eliminate foods from your diet that make the blood acidic.

The major acid-forming foods in our diets include animal proteins,[15] soft drinks, sugar, salt, caffeine and alcohol. Americans consume too much of all

---

[14] Fad Diets Versus Dietary Guidelines, American Institute for Cancer Research, 02/11/02:12.

[15] Advocates of high-protein diets will claim that animal protein has no effect on bone loss. To support this claim, they will quote the work of Herta Spencer, who published two oft-quoted studies. These were badly flawed and biased studies. Not surprisingly,

these products. In the case of sodium, we get most of it not from table salt, but indirectly in packaged and processed foods. In fact, dairy products and processed meat are the biggest sources of sodium in the American diet.

High acidity is bad for a number of reasons. First, high acid levels make our bodies more cancer friendly by reducing the delivery of oxygen to cells. In addition, cancer cells love highly acidic environments and do not do well in healthy, alkaline environments. Second, a highly acidic environment disrupts the function of enzymes and the digestion of food. Undigested food gets passed into the colon and sits there, rotting, and this can lead to toxic buildups and a number of health problems. The average American stores 4 to 22 pounds of old (sometimes decades old!) fecal matter in their colons. John Wayne had almost 44 pounds of undigested sludge in his colon. Elvis had over 20 pounds.[16] Crayons people have swallowed as children have later been discovered in their 60-year old colons! Third, when blood becomes too acidic, our bodies pull calcium from our bones and teeth to neutralize the acid and this contributes to bone loss, or osteoporosis. The body also pulls water from cells to neutralize high acid levels and this leads to cell dehydration, which many experts believe is the number one cause of premature aging.

The way Americans consume antacids is a reflection of just how acidic our diet has become; but taking a calcium pill to neutralize high acid levels is treating a symptom. If you want to eliminate the problem, you'll have to radically cut back on acidic foods.

By continually eating foods which cause high blood acid levels, we put our bodies in a state of constantly having to neutralize this acid by using the calcium stored up in our bones. Animal proteins are one of the most acid-forming foods in existence and because of our high-protein diets, the biggest cause of high acid levels. One reason dairy products are poor choices for calcium is because they contain excessively high amounts of protein. Cow's milk has over three times more protein than human mother's milk. It was, after all, designed for a calf that will weigh over 300 pounds within a year of its birth.

When you consume dairy products, the calcium simply passes through your body and ends up in the toilet – and your blood is even more acidic because of the protein. Low-fat dairy products are highest in protein, so you may lower your fat intake, but you will raise your blood acid level and this will contribute to bone loss. Skim milk, for example, contains almost twice the amount of protein as

---

one was paid for by the National Dairy Council (Spencer H. Effect of a high protein (meat) intake on calcium metabolism in man. Am J Clin Nutr. 1978 Dec;31(12):2167-80) and the other by the National Livestock and Meat Board (Spencer H. Further studies of the effect of a high protein diet as meat on calcium metabolism. Am J Clin Nutr. 1983 Jun;37(6):924-9).
[16] See www.thedoctorwithin.com Chapter on Enzymes.

whole milk. And because of the high sodium content of dairy products, they provide a double-boost to your acid levels.

In short, consuming dairy products turns out to be the worst possible way to build strong bones. You don't need the sodium, the fat, the acidic proteins, the cholesterol – and you don't need the excess calcium, which can result in painful kidney stones.

The cause of osteoporosis is *not* a lack of calcium in the diet, regardless of the advertising from the dairy industry. Populations that consume the highest amount of calcium have the highest rates of osteoporosis. In fact, the more calcium they consume, the higher their rates of osteoporosis. Conversely, the countries with the *least* amount of calcium consumption have the lowest rates of osteoporosis. Obviously, something else is going on because it's not a lack of calcium that's causing osteoporosis.

What gives? Although Americans are swimming in calcium, the World Health Organization has yet to document a single case of calcium deficiency anywhere in the world.[17] In fact, there has not been a single recorded case of calcium deficiency of a dietary origin in the history of the entire planet.[18] Yet, the dairy industry tells Americans they have a calcium deficiency.

The problem, of course, is that the dairy industry has set U.S. standards for calcium consumption sky high through lobbying efforts. The calcium scare that has been going on in this country is, without question, the biggest nutritional swindle ever conceived. If you think this is an outrageous statement, then show me a single case of calcium deficiency of a dietary origin. (If you're thinking of rickets, that disease is caused by a lack of vitamin D, not a lack of calcium.)

You'll hear health authorities say that women should get between 1,000 and 1,500 mg of calcium per day, while men should get 1,000 mg per day. What would these health authorities say to men and women throughout the world who get only 200 mg a day – and have bones much stronger than Americans? In fact, 70-year-old women in Third World countries who have nursed multiple children have bones stronger than most 40-year-old women in this country. And they get their calcium from plant foods, not dairy products.

Osteoporosis is *not* genetic and you don't have to suffer bone loss if you change your exercise and eating habits. When people say it runs in the family, it simply means the family has led a sedentary lifestyle over generations. Many women, including Dr. Ruth Heidrich (interviewed in the film *Eating*), increased

---

[17] The Pritikin Program for Diet & Exercise, Nathan Pritikin, M.D., p. 44.

[18] McDougall's Medicine, John A. McDougall, M.D., p. 70; The McDougall Program, John A. McDougall, M.D., p. 48, Calcium Requirements in man: a critical review, C. Paterson, Postgrad Med J. 54:244, 1978; The human requirement of calcium: should low intakes be supplemented? A. Walker, Am J. Clin Nutr, 25:518, 1972; Symposium on human calcium requirements: Council on Foods and Nutrition, JAMA 185:588, 1963; Modern Nutrition in Health and Disease, 5th ed, Goodhart and Shils, 1973, p. 274.

their bone mass during and after menopause without dairy products or hormone replacement therapy.

Bones are just like muscles. The single best thing you can do to prevent (and reverse) osteoporosis is to start exercising your bones, because *a lack of physical activity is the primary cause of osteoporosis.*

Acidic diets will cause bone loss, but not as rapidly as a lack of exercise. People who argue that acidic diets are the primary cause of bone loss have a big flaw in their argument: There are lots of meat-eaters with strong bones. This is because their activity levels strengthen their bones, despite a bad diet. Also, obese women and men never get osteoporosis because they get lots of weight-bearing exercise just carrying their bodies around, regardless of their diet and calcium intake. Lighter women and men have increased chances of osteoporosis simply because their bodies don't have enough weight – unless they run or jog to add stress to their bones. In other words, lighter men and women need to engage in weight-bearing activity in order to strengthen their bones. Swimming is a good illustration of how a lack of stress on bones plays out – because runners have higher femur bone densities than swimmers.

It's never been proven that a plant-based diet alone can reverse osteoporosis. It has been proven that exercise reverses osteoporosis. In fact, NASA regularly reverses osteoporosis in astronauts when they return to earth with an exercise program, not a change in diet. In fact, on that basis alone, exercise is the most proven way to reverse bone loss. (Osteoporosis is a potentially huge problem for long-term space flight because, due to the lack of gravity, NASA is afraid they'd end up with boneless astronauts!)

There are no studies, that I am aware of, which factor both exercise and diet into the equation to determine which is most important. There are, however, hundreds – if not thousands – of studies which show far more dramatic differences in bone density between those who get regular exercise and those who do not.[19] And those differences are gigantic compared to studies that show differences in bone density between people eating different diets. On that basis alone, one has to conclude that exercise is the most important factor affecting bone density. The effect of weight-bearing activity on bone density are extraordinarily well-documented and have consistently shown the same results over decades, regardless of diet.

---

[19] JAMA. 2002;288:2300-2306 (41% difference in hip fractures between those women who exercised and those who did not); Aloia, J., Exercise and skeletal health. Journal of American Geriatric Society 29:104, 1981., Smith, E., Physical activity and calcium modalities for bone mineral increase in aged women. Med Sci, Sports Exercise 13:60, 1981, Gymnastics Strengthens Girls' Bones: Study Journal of Pediatrics 2002;141:211-216, Journal of Pediatrics 2002;141:211-216, Smith, E.L., 1982. Exercise for prevention of osteoporosis: A review. The Physician and Sportsmedicine 10(3):72-82.

A recent study showed that varying levels of calcium intake, ranging from 500 mg a day to 1800 mg a day, had *absolutely no effect on bone strength*. It was the *exercise* women got that was the key determinant in building strong bones.[20]

We're worrying about vitamin A and vitamin D and getting enough calcium – all these worries – but no one is worrying about getting enough exercise. Our worries are solely the result of advertising by the dairy industry and the government, which sponsors the dairy industry. To think you can just eat your way out of osteoporosis or take calcium supplements is ridiculous.

Don't worry about calcium. Do worry about exercise. We have this crazy idea that somehow cows produce calcium. They're simply storage systems for the calcium they get from the plants they eat. Calcium comes from the earth – like all other minerals – and plant foods are the best place not only to get calcium, but all the other minerals the body needs. Get your calcium from inexpensive plant foods like the rest of the world does. Plant foods will keep your blood acid level in balance because they're alkaline, not acidic. Like protein, calcium is found in all plant foods and the amounts will easily supply the requirements of growing children and mature adults.

Calcium from plant foods is more easily absorbed by bone than calcium from dairy products and unlike dairy, calcium from plants comes in a disease-fighting, low-fat, high-fiber package. Cut back or eliminate all foods that contribute to high acid levels. Diet and exercise are the keys to preventing and reversing osteoporosis. A change in diet will prevent bone loss and exercise is the *only* way to build strong bones.

To demonstrate just how much calcium is in plant foods, a quick comparison of the calcium content of dairy products versus plant foods is shown below.

---

[20] Study: Exercise Important for Strong Bones, AP, 6/9/04.

Calcium in Milligrams per 100 Calories

Arugula	1,300
Bok choy	1,055
Turnip greens	921
Watercress	800
Collard greens	559
Mustard greens	490
Spinach	450
Broccoli	387
Romaine lettuce	257
Swiss cheese	250
Milk (2-percent)	245
Green onions	240
Okra	213
Cabbage	196
Whole milk	190
Sesame seeds	170
Cheddar cheese	179
American cheese	160
Soybeans	134
Cucumber	108

Surprised to see all those plant foods have more calcium than two percent milk? Of course, you're probably saying, "But I would have to eat so much more spinach or kale to get adequate calcium." This is not true because individuals on plant-based diets generally eat as many calories as people eating the standard American diet. In other words, you can get all the calcium you need from the original source of calcium, without getting it second-hand in a package of saturated fat and cholesterol.

Another way to look at it is to compare the calcium content of plant foods to mother's milk:

Calcium content of foods (per 100-gram portion)

Human Breast Milk - 33

Almonds - 234
Amaranth - 267
Apricots (dried) - 67
Artichokes - 51
Beans (can: pinto, black) - 135
Beet greens (cooked) - 99
Blackeye peas - 55
Bran - 70
Broccoli (raw) - 48
Brussels Sprouts - 36
Buckwheat - 114
Cabbage (raw) - 49
Carrot (raw) - 37
Cashew nuts - 38
Cauliflower (cooked) - 42
Swiss Chard (raw) - 88
Chickpeas (garbanzos) - 150
Collards (raw leaves) - 250
Cress (raw) - 81
Dandelion greens - 187
Endive - 81
Escarole - 81
Figs (dried) - 126
Filberts (Hazelnuts) - 209
Kale (raw leaves) - 249
Kale (cooked leaves) - 187
Leeks - 52
Lettuce (lt. green) - 35

Lettuce (dark green) - 68
Molasses (dark-213 cal.) - 684
Mustard Green (raw) - 183
Mustard Green (cooked) - 138
Okra (raw or cooked) - 92
Olives - 61
Orange (Florida) - 43
Parsley - 203
Peanuts (roasted & salted) - 74
Peas (boiled) - 56
Pistachio nuts - 131
Potato Chips - 40
Raisins - 62
Rhubarb (cooked) - 78
Sauerkraut - 36
Sesame Seeds - 1160
Squash (Butternut) - 40
Soybeans - 60
Sugar (Brown) - 85
Tofu - 85
Spinach (raw) - 93
Sunflower seeds - 120
Sweet Potatoes (baked) - 40
Turnips (cooked) - 35
Turnip Greens (raw) - 246
Turnip Greens (boiled) - 184
Water Cress – 151

Genetics

"Genes load the gun. Lifestyle pulls the trigger." - Caldwell Esselstyn, M.D.

People like to blame diseases on their genes, but only a very small percentage of our major diseases are caused by genetics. If genes were important, we would simply not have the explosion of diseases that characterizes the American health landscape today.

We are all born with a matrix of genes which can make us more or less susceptible to a wide range of diseases. The "bad" genes, however, are almost always dormant and do not become active players unless the right conditions set them off. A bad diet and lifestyle will create those conditions. A healthy diet and lifestyle will keep bad genes quiet and they will never trigger a disease.

There are also people who like to credit their good genes for their longevity. The Okinawans, for example, are known to have the longest disability-free life expectancy of any people in the world and many Okinawans like to give credit to their genetic makeup. Yet, all you have to do is look at younger Okinawans living near American military bases. Unlike their parents, they have adopted the American fast food culture and as a result, they have Japan's highest rates of obesity, heart disease and premature death. Also, when Okinawans migrate to America and adopt the American diet and lifestyle, their rates of disease and longevity soon match the American rates.

Most people see genes as immutable and unchanging – you're either doomed or saved by your genetic makeup. We're finding out now that this is not at all true, and that diet and lifestyle can directly affect how your genes are expressed.[1]

Dr. Dean Ornish took a small group of men with early stage prostate cancer and put them on a plant-based diet coupled with exercise. In just three months, the men had changes in activity in about 500 genes, including 48 that were turned on by the diet and exercise – and 452 that were turned off![2]

Cigarette smoking alters the pattern of genes expressed in cells lining the airways. Some 97 genes were expressed differently than in people who had never smoked.[3] A gene for a protein that regulates cholesterol is potentially lethal for smokers in terms of heart disease. But if you give up smoking and change to a healthy diet and lifestyle, the genetic predisposition for heart disease can be eliminated.[4]

Women with the BRCA1 and BRCA2 genes have up to an 80 percent risk of developing breast cancer IF they have a strong family history of breast cancer. Women carrying these genes who do not have a strong family history have only a ten percent chance of developing breast cancer – or about the same as if they didn't have the bad gene at all. That's a whopping 800 percent variation in outcome – all depending on family history. What does family history mean? It means a history of diet and lifestyle that awakens this gene.

---

[1] This is called nutrigenomics. For more information, see "Nutrigenomics in public health nutrition: short-term perspectives", Chavez A, Munoz de Chavez M, European Journal of Clinical Nutrition. 57(Suppl. 1)97-100; "Nutrigenomics: Goals and Perspectives.", Müller M, Kersten S., Nature Reviews Genetics 4. 315 -322; "Nutritional genomics-"Nutrigenomics", Trayhurn P., British Journal Nutrition. 89:1-2.

[2] As reported in MSNBC, June 16, 2008; www.msnbc.msn.com/id/25199024/.

[3] Avrum Spira, et al. Effects of cigarette smoke on the human airway epithelial cell transcriptome. PNAS July 6, 2004 vol. 101 no. 27 10143-10148.

[4] As reported by Ann Underwood, Jerry Adler. Diet and Genes. Newsweek. 1/24/05.

That diet and lifestyle have a huge impact can be seen in the fact that women carrying the mutated BRCA1 gene are 60 percent less likely to have breast cancer if they were breast fed for more than a year.[5] It's also been found that women carrying these genes can reduce their risks of breast cancer by up to 65 percent simply by losing weight.[6] Conversely, it's been found that gaining 10 pounds increased their risk of developing cancer. If you start putting all the healthy diet and lifestyle factors together, you can put these genes to sleep quite simply.

Even without this bad gene, women who just have a family history of breast cancer feel hopeless and are opting for double mastectomies as a prophylactic measure. What they don't realize is that having both breasts removed does not reduce their risks of getting uterine cancer, liver cancer, lymph cancer, or a host of other cancers. And there are better ways to reduce their risks of getting breast cancer, regardless of family history.

The latest theory regarding colon cancer is that it's one of the most commonly inherited cancer syndromes known, and the medical intelligentsia has developed an elaborate explanation for this so-called genetically based disease. What they fail to mention in their explanation is that colon cancer was virtually unknown 100 years ago, and yet it's now the single leading cancer in men and women combined. Genes don't change across generations in the short span of 100 years. Only diet and lifestyle change that rapidly.

A recent study[7] has shown that genetic links to cancers have been greatly exaggerated and, in fact, genetics is far less important to cancer than past studies (and headlines) have led people to believe. The study analyzed hundreds of other studies that claimed to have "discovered" genes that cause cancer. It found out that of 240 claimed associations between genes and cancer risk, in fact only two genes actually had any significant correlation at all, or less than one percent![8]

Another problem is the words "association" and "correlation" because these are statistical artifacts which do not show causation – they in no way demonstrate that a specific gene or genes will cause cancer. The correlations between genetics and cancer were exaggerated. Why? In my opinion, it was probably an attempt to elevate the importance of genes in the hope of getting research money because drug companies are targeting gene therapy as the new frontier for developing magic bullet drugs. They can then show success with these drugs by using

---

[5] Journal of the National Cancer Institute, July 21, 2004.

[6] As reported by the BBC, August 19, 2005.

[7] As reported in "Many studies needed to tie genes to cancer," Reuters, 12/30/08. Lead authors were John Ioannidis of the University of Ioannina School of Medicine and Paolo Vineis of Imperial College London, for those who wish to look it up. The study had not yet been published at the time of this writing.

[8] The study did not examine the BRCA1 or BRCA2 genetic link.

relative (rubber) numbers. The same gene-disease link exaggeration is now happening across the board with other diseases, e.g., Alzheimer's.[9]

The problem, of course, is that magic bullet treatments have never been successful in treating cancer – or any other long-term degenerative disease – and never will be, due to the nature of these diseases.

If genes were that important, we would simply not have the explosion of diseases that characterizes the American health landscape, i.e., genetic makeup did not create the mess we're in today. Many people are genetically susceptible to adult-onset diabetes, for example. If they eat a diet full of animal and refined foods, it is a virtual certainty they will get diabetes. If they do not eat these foods, they simply will not get diabetes, regardless of their genes. In fact, all populations have people who are genetically predisposed to certain diseases. But some populations never get these diseases due to their diet and lifestyle. So despite these genetic predispositions, you can overcome genetic weaknesses through diet. And if you never ate these harmful foods, you would never even know about your genetic predispositions. Heart disease and our common cancers were unknown in many countries throughout the world – until the American diet was introduced to them.

A typical response by cardiologists to the question, "How can I prevent heart disease?" is to answer, "Pick the right parents." Unfortunately, most cardiologists know more about bypass surgeries than they know about the cause of heart disease. In fact, it's almost 100 percent caused by diet.

Genes are important, but often they give us a false sense of security. For example, a small percentage of the population has the ability to get rid of cholesterol very efficiently. Thus, they can eat all the meat they want and keep their total cholesterol levels below 150. (And those people pushing high-fat diets will point to these people and argue that meat has nothing to do with cardiovascular disease.) This is true for only for a very tiny part of the population, who are genetically blessed this way. On the other hand, heart disease is only one of many diseases that have been linked to animal and refined foods and the ability to jettison large quantities of cholesterol from their bodies certainly does not keep them safe from these other diseases.

Genes do matter, but people gamble on them, hoping their good genes will save them from a lifetime of nutritional abuse. At the other end of the spectrum, some people think they're doomed because they have a family history of a disease. Neither case is accurate and to bet your life on your genes will be the biggest gamble you'll ever take.

Don't count on grandpa's genes to save you from a self-destructive lifestyle. Most of us have nutritional time bombs ticking inside of us. If you're smart,

---

[9] Kavvoura FK, et al. Evaluation of the potential excess of statistically significant findings in published genetic association studies: application to Alzheimer's disease. Am J Epidemiol. 2008 Oct 15;168(8):855-65.

you'll play the odds and change your diet to improve the quality of your life so you can, in fact, grow old gracefully, with dignity, and without a regimen of debilitating drugs.

Supplementation

You cannot put nature in a pill.

People love their supplements, almost as much as they hate their vegetables. What most are trying to do is make up for their bad eating habits, but that is simply not possible because isolated synthetic supplements are weak substitutes for the vibrant strength of the integrated micronutrients you get from whole plant foods in their natural states.

When you peruse the newspapers, you will see reports of studies which show that this vitamin or that vitamin had no effect in combating a particular disease. What you have to pay attention to is that – without exception – these studies are looking at the synthetic version of the vitamin – a pill – which has no magic. It's lost its mojo. What you will never see is a study which states that a vitamin taken in its natural state (in food) had no effect on a disease. Natural vitamins always have a positive effect!

One of the most famous studies showing how impotent supplements are had to do with beta-carotene supplements actually *increasing* the risk for lung cancer in heavy smokers.[10] Vitamin A or beta-carotene supplements may also interfere with the absorption of carotenoids such as lutein and lycopene, and this interference can increase the risks of developing cancer.[11] You will never find this to be the case with natural sources of beta-carotene found in food.

Recently it was reported that after spending millions of dollars, scientists found that vitamins E and selenium *synthetic supplements* are useless for combating prostate cancer.[12] A number of other recent studies using synthetic supplements came to the same conclusion.[13] The problem is that supplements

---

[10] The effect of vitamin E and beta carotene on the incidence of lung cancer and other cancers in male smokers, The Alpha-Tocopherol, Beta Carotene Cancer Prevention Study Group, NEJM, 1994 Apr 14;330(15):1029-35; Omenn GS, Effects of a combination of beta carotene and vitamin A on lung cancer and cardiovascular disease, N Engl J Med. 1996 May 2;334(18):1150-5.

[11] Mayne ST. Beta-carotene, carotenoids, and disease prevention in humans. FASEB. 1996;10(7):690-701.

[12] See The SELECT Prostate Cancer Prevention Trial at http://www.cancer.gov/clinicaltrials/digestpage/SELECT

[13] Jennifer Lin, et al., Vitamins C and E and Beta Carotene Supplementation and Cancer Risk: A Randomized Controlled Trial. J. Natl. Cancer Inst..2008; 0: djn438 v1-23;

alone won't do a thing about cancer. You have to change your overall diet and lifestyle. Supplements may help, but taking them alone without changing your diet and lifestyle won't be of much help.

The findings of such studies are not surprising because synthetic supplements – concentrated and *isolated* forms of vitamins and minerals – throw the body off balance because nowhere can such concentrations be found in nature. And the body has been trained to expect what comes from nature.

People always assume that more is better. When it comes to supplements, however, that is usually not the case. Vitamin A supplements have been shown to cause a one in 57 chance of birth defects when taken by pregnant women, as well as increasing the risk of hip fractures in older women.[14] Iron supplementation has been shown to cause a fatal liver disease.[15] Magnesium supplementation has been shown to increase the risk of heart attacks and sudden death, particularly among people with heart disease.[16] Zinc *and* iron supplements may also increase the risk of death from heart disease.[17]

Folic acid supplementation has been shown to reduce the risk of birth defects, but it was recently discovered it also increased the risks of colon cancer.[18] It's also been found that getting enough folic acid may keep tumors from starting by repairing DNA errors, but getting too much may feed tumors once they start.[19]

There is also controversy about taking synthetic antioxidant supplementation during radiation treatments with reports showing they interfered with the treatment's "effectiveness."[20] Although the dust is still settling on this

---

Vitamins C and E and Beta Carotene Again Fail to Reduce Cancer Risk in Randomized Controlled Trial. J Natl Cancer Inst 2008 0: djn501v1-1.

[14] Michaelsson K., Serum retinol levels and the risk of fracture, N Engl J Med. 2003 Jan 23;348(4):287-94; Dolk HM, Dietary vitamin A and teratogenic risk: European Teratology Society discussion paper, Eur J Obstet Gynecol Reprod Biol. 1999 Mar;83(1):31-6; Rothman KJ. Teratogenicity of high vitamin A intake. N Engl J Med. 1995 Nov 23;333(21):1369-73.

[15] Schumann K., Safety aspects of iron in food, Ann Nutr Metab. 2001;45(3):91-101.

[16] Galloe AM, Influence of oral magnesium supplementation on cardiac events among survivors of an acute myocardial infarction, BMJ, 1993 Sep 4;307(6904):585-7.

[17] Galloe AM, Influence of oral magnesium supplementation on cardiac events among survivors of an acute myocardial infarction, BMJ, 1993 Sep 4;307(6904):585-7; Black MR, Zinc supplements and serum lipids in young adult white males, Am J Clin Nutr. 1988 Jun;47(6):970-5.

[18] See Fortifying foods with the vitamin has reduced certain birth defects but may have raised rates of colon cancer, Los Angeles Times, August 6, 2007.

[19] Ulrich C., Folate and cancer prevention: a closer look at a complex picture, Am J Clin Nut; 2007; 86(2)271-273.

[20] Bairati I, Meyer F, Jobin E, Gélinas M, Fortin A, Nabid A, Brochet F, Têtu B., Antioxidant vitamins supplementation and mortality: a randomized trial in head and neck cancer patients, Int J Cancer. 2006;119(9):2221-4; Lawenda B et al. Should supplemental antioxidant administration be avoided during chemotherapy and radiation

controversy, what is clear is that the adverse reactions were only experienced by those who still smoked. But the bottom line is that the micronutrients from whole foods will always help, even with smokers.

The examples are really endless and they all point to the same thing: Artificial, synthetic supplements throw the body off balance and can result in serious and unexpected side effects. Natural foods in their natural packages keep the body in balance.

You will no doubt run across testimonials regarding initial positive results from taking many supplements (from herbal extracts to mango juice). These can be ascribed to the placebo effect. Over the long-term, however, it has not been shown that supplements work – unless you take care of the fundamentals of diet and lifestyle. That is to say, if you take wonder supplement #1 and you're eating hamburgers all day, that supplement may make you feel much better (despite the hamburgers), but once the placebo effect wears off, you will come crashing down with the reality of your diet.

Synthetic supplements have their place in deficiency diseases, such as scurvy, which is caused by a deficiency of vitamin C. But cancer is not a deficiency disease of a single nutrient[21] and cannot be healed with the application of a single or even multiple nutrients, particularly in synthetic form. A vitamin's benefit, in other words, will become apparent only if people are not getting enough of it. Supplementation can have a place in the short-term healing of diseases, but in the long-term, they will cause problems.

With regard to short-term supplementation, if you are currently undergoing conventional treatments you will no doubt need supplementation of some sort because of the devastating effects of chemo on the body. However, many of the most common herbal supplements have the potential to interact with cancer drugs in negative ways, so you need to tell your oncologist about what you are doing.[22] You should also seek advice about supplements from a clinic which has

---

therapy?, J Natl Canc Inst. 2008;100:773–783; Meyer F, Bairati I, Jobin E, Gélinas M, Fortin A, Nabid A, Têtu B., Acute adverse effects of radiation therapy and local recurrence in relation to dietary and plasma beta carotene and alpha tocopherol in head and neck cancer patients., Nutr Cancer. 2007;59(1):29-35; Meyer F, Bairati I, Fortin A, Gélinas M, Nabid A, Brochet F, Têtu B., Interaction between antioxidant vitamin supplementation and cigarette smoking during radiation therapy in relation to long-term effects on recurrence and mortality: a randomized trial among head and neck cancer patients. Int J Cancer. 2008;122(7):1679-83.

[21] Proponents of laetrile will argue that cancer is caused by a deficiency of vitamin B-17, but B-17 supplementation is neither the cause nor the cure for cancer. For more on this, see the book, Healing Cancer From Inside Out by Mike Anderson.

[22] In one study, researchers found that nearly half of women being treated for breast and gynecologic cancers used some type of herbal or vitamin supplement and of those, half did not inform their doctors. See Journal of Clinical Oncology Vol. 22, No. 4: 671-677.

experience using them with people who either are currently undergoing conventional treatments or have undergone such treatments.

To be sure, we have nutritional deficiencies in the area of micronutrients, but our bodies work as a symphony and the absorption of micronutrients from whole plant foods will orchestrate the healing of the body in a way that single or multiple magic bullet supplements cannot.

Raw vs. Cooked Foods

There is considerably controversy between "raw foodists" and those who like their foods cooked (or a combination of raw and cooked foods). In *Essential Dietary Guidelines*, I recommend that at least half of your food be uncooked, primarily because cooked foods tend to contain fewer phytochemicals and antioxidants than fresh, uncooked foods.

However, that is not always the case. For example, cooking vegetables increases the content of soluble fiber, which helps fight diseases in many different ways. On the other hand, cooking decreases the content of insoluble fiber, which fights diseases by binding and excreting carcinogens, excess hormones and other toxins.[23] Cooking fights cancer by destroying some of the pesticides present in non-organic produce, but cooking also destroys enzymes that have beneficial effects in digesting foods. Cooking dark green leafy vegetables may destroy half of the antioxidant carotenoids,[24] yet at the same time, cooking may double carotenoid bioavailability.[25]

Raw garlic may be healthier than cooked due to an enzyme called alliinase, which produces a DNA-protecting compound called allicin when chewed in your mouth. When cooked, you absorb little or none of this compound.[26]

An enzyme called myrosinase is produced when chewing raw broccoli. This enzyme can rev up your liver's ability to detoxify carcinogens. Cooking completely deactivates this enzyme, while steaming will produce only a third as much of this enzyme as eating broccoli raw.[27]

Eating cruciferous vegetables (e.g. kale, collards, broccoli, etc.) allows one to absorb two cancer-fighting phytonutrients called isothiocyantes and indoles. With raw cruciferous vegetables, you increase your intake of isothiocyantes, but with cooked, you increase your intake of indoles.

Cruciferous vegetables are the best source of a cancer-fighting nutrient called sulforaphane. In one study, the amount of sulforaphane actually absorbed by

---

[23] Plant Foods in Human Nutrition 55(2000):207.
[24] Journal of the National Cancer Institute 82(1990):282.
[25] Journal of Nutrition 128(1998):913.
[26] Journal of Nutrition 131(2001):1054.
[27] Nutrition and Cancer 38(2000):168.

human test subjects was ten times higher with raw broccoli than with cooked broccoli.[28]

Raw foodists claim that a raw food diet is healthier, but not for the reasons they provide, which range from eating "live food" or because of the "life force," "living enzymes," or "nerve energy" in the food. What it boils down to is that foods which can be eaten raw (primarily fruits and vegetables) have enormously higher nutrient values, per calorie, than the foods that either have to be, or usually are, cooked. [29]

The bottom line? Eat your greens. At least half of your food should be uncooked and the more the better because of the higher nutrient content, per calorie, of low fat fruits and vegetables.

Soy and Breast Cancer

There has been a lot of controversy over soy and breast cancer. Studies which claim soy increases the risk of breast cancer are based on looking at *refined* soy products and many of these studies are very questionable in the first place.[30] There is no credible evidence linking the whole organic soy bean (endamame) with increased breast (or other) cancer risks. In fact, studies point to decreased cancer risks when consuming whole organic soy beans.[31]

---

[28] J Agric Food Chem 2008;56:10505-9.

[29] For an excellent article examining the controversy of raw vs. cooked foods, see William Harris, M.D., www.vegsource.com/harris/raw_vs_cooked.htm.

[30] For a review of some of the fallacious arguments and agendas of soy-bashers, see www.eatkind.net/wholesoystory.htm.

[31] Messina M, Barnes S: The role of soy products in reducing risk of cancer. J Natl Cancer Inst 1991, 83:541-546; Lee HP, Gourley L, Duffy SW, Esteve J, Lee J, Day NE: Dietary effects on breast-cancer risk in Singapore. Lancet 1991, 337:1197-2000; Barnes S, Grubbs C, Setchell KD, Carlson J: Soybeans inhibit mammary tumors in models of breast cancer; Prog Clin Biol Res 1990, 347::239-253; Messina MJ, Loprinzi CL: Soy for breast cancer survivors: a critical review of the literature. J Nutr 2001, 131:3095S-108S; Jefferson WN, Newbold RR: Potential endocrine-modulating effects of various phytoestrogens in the diet. Nutrition 2000, 16:658-662; An J, Tzagarakis-Foster C, Scharschmidt TC, Lomri N, Leitman DC: Estrogen Receptor beta -Selective Transcriptional Activity and Recruitment of Coregulators by Phytoestrogens. J Biol Chem 2001, 276:17808-17814; Zava DT, Duwe G: Estrogenic and antiproliferative properties of genistein and other flavonoids in human breast cancer cells in vitro. Nutr Cancer 1997, 27:31-40; Wu AH, Yu MC, Tseng CC, Pike MC: Epidemiology of soy exposures and breast cancer risk. Br J Cancer 2008, 98:9-14; Messina M, McCaskill-Stevens W, Lampe JW: Addressing the soy and breast cancer relationship: review, commentary, and workshop proceedings. J Natl Cancer Inst 2006, 98:1275-1284; Yonemoto RH: Breast cancer in Japan and United States: epidemiology, hormone

Researchers have theorized that natural soy compounds called isoflavones, which have weak estrogen-like effects, could lower breast cancer risk by binding to estrogen receptors in breast tissue and blocking the cancer-promoting effects of the hormone.

But many experts wonder that with its estrogen-like effects, it may promote the growth of estrogen-sensitive cancers (breast and prostate), especially for those people who already have cancer.[32] While soy isoflavones do function as weak estrogens in animal and test tube studies, most of these experiments use unrealistically large amounts of isoflavones – equivalent to *five to sixteen times the amount commonly consumed in Asia*. And this is the basic problem with studies linking soy with breast cancer.

In fact, studies point to decreased cancer risks when consuming moderate amounts of *whole* soy beans.[33] One recent study showed a 13 percent drop in PSA after just one month of adding two ounces of soy each day to their diet.[34] Two ounces a day, by the way, is the typical amount of soy eaten in traditional Chinese and Japanese diets.[35] Breast and prostate cancer rates are four to six times lower in Japan and China than Western countries and laboratory studies

---

receptors, pathology, and survival. Arch Surg 1980, 115:1056-1062; Morrison AS, Lowe CR, MacMahon B, Ravnihar B, Yuasa S: Some international differences in treatment and survival in breast cancer. Int J Cancer 1976, 18:269-273; Murkies A, Dalais FS, Briganti EM, Burger HG, Healy DL, Wahlqvist ML, Davis SR: Phytoestrogens and breast cancer in postmenopausal women: a case control study. Menopause 2000, 7:289-296; De Lemos M: Safety issues of soy phytoestrogens in breast cancer patients. J Clin Oncol 2002, 20:3040-1; Murphy PA, Song T, Buseman G, Barua K, Beecher GR, Trainer D, Holden J: Isoflavones in retail and institutional soy foods. J Agric Food Chem 1999, 47:2697-2704; Boker LK, Van der Schouw YT, De Kleijn MJ, Jacques PF, Grobbee DE, Peeters PH: Intake of dietary phytoestrogens by Dutch women. J Nutr 2002, 132:1319-1328; Takashima N, Miyanaga N, Komiya K, More M, Akaza H: Blood isoflavone levels during intake of a controlled hospital diet. J Nutr Sci Vitaminol (Tokyo) 2004, 50:246-252; Brzezinski A, Adlercreutz H, Shaoul R, Rösler R, Shmueli A, Tanos V, Schenker JG: Short-term effect of phytoestrogen-rich diet on postmenopausal women. Menopause 1997, 4:89-94.

[32] Newbold R. Uterine adenocarcinoma in mice treated neonatally with genistein. Cancer Res. 2001 Jun 1;61(11):4325-8; Cassileth BR, Vickers AJ. Soy: an anticancer agent in wide use despite some troubling data. Cancer Invest. 2003;21(5):817-8.

[33] Messina MJ, Barnes S. The role of soy products in reducing risk of cancer. J Natl Cancer Inst 1991;83:541-6.

[34] See Dalias, F. Urology, September 2004; vol 64, pp 510-515; Kumar, N. Prostate, May 2004; vol 59; pp 141-147.

[35] Nagata C, Takatsuka N, Kurisu Y, Shimizu H. Decreased serum total cholesterol concentration is associated with high intake of soy products in Japanese men and women. J Nutr. 1998 Feb;128(2):209-13.

have shown that isoflavone from soy can inhibit the growth of both breast and prostate cancer tissues.[36]

A recent analysis has concluded that soy isoflavones' estrogen-like effects are probably too weak to have any significant consequence on breast tissue in healthy women, even breast cancer survivors.[37] As the authors stated, "Overall, there is little clinical evidence to suggest that isoflavones will increase breast cancer risk in healthy women or worsen the prognosis of breast cancer patients."

Given all the controversy, however, you may not be at ease with soy, even the whole, organic bean eaten in moderate amounts. There is a very easy solution to this dilemma: Eliminate soy from your diet. It's as simple as that because there are many other foods to choose from on a plant-based diet that will give you what you need without having to consume soy.

[36] Adlercreutz H. Phyto-oestrogens and cancer. Lancet Oncol. 2002 Jun;3(6):364-73.
[37] Mark J Messina, Charles E Wood. Soy isoflavones, estrogen therapy, and breast cancer risk: analysis and commentary. Nutrition Journal 2008, 7:17 (3 June 2008).

RAVE Diet Guidelines

The RAVE Diet Food Pyramid

Let's take a brief tour of the RAVE Diet food pyramid.

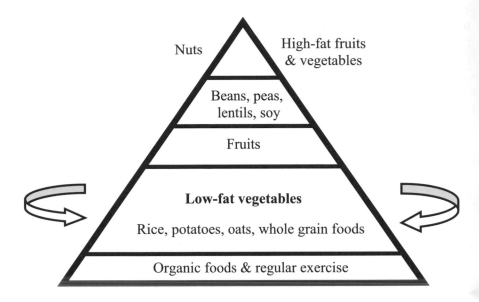

RAVE foods are the only foods that contain both fiber and cancer-fighting nutrients *in the same package*. At the top are foods with a high fat to fiber ratio. As you move down the pyramid, the amount of fat decreases, relative to the amount of fiber.

At the very top are foods such as nuts, seeds and high-fat fruits and vegetables, like avocados and olives. Great foods, but over 80 percent fat, so go easy on them. (This includes nut butters.)

The higher protein foods tend to be beans, peas, lentils and soy. These are near the top of the pyramid because they are still high in fat content, so you need to watch the proportions. And you don't need to eat these foods to get protein. Both protein and calcium are found throughout the pyramid and you'll get more than adequate amounts of both – as well as all other essential nutrients – by just eating any variety of these foods.

Vegetables and fruits are the two most important food groups for fighting diseases and keeping you looking and feeling young. Optimally, your diet should really be centered on *low-fat vegetables*. In fact, low-fat vegetables can occupy a much larger portion of the pyramid if you want, depending on your food preferences. Leafy green vegetables, for example, can give you practically everything you need in terms of nutrients – that's how good they are. In fact, calorie-for-calorie, green vegetables are the most nutritious foods on the planet.

At the base of the pyramid are rice, potatoes and whole grain foods. Use these as meat substitutes to fill you up. Avoid white rice because the fiber, vitamins and other nutrients have been removed. Choose brown rice instead (or another *whole* grain rice) and always eat potatoes with the skin. Potatoes are 1 percent fat, brown rice is 6 percent fat, wild rice is 3 percent fat, barley and bulgur are both 3 percent fat. All of the whole-wheat grains are under 10 percent fat. Compare that with typical (non-fried) servings of rib steak (78%), chicken (54%), turkey (42%) or Atlantic salmon (54%), and you can see where we're going with this.

You'll hear some people say to eat fruits and low-fat vegetables exclusively and avoid "starchy" foods at the bottom of the pyramid, as well as the high-fat foods at the top of the pyramid. This is good advice, but not everyone can eat like this and feel satisfied. Rice, potatoes, corn and other whole grain foods serve as "filler foods" because they are satisfying and fill you up. In their natural forms, these foods are very low in fat (potatoes are only one percent fat) and rich in nutrients. As you start out on the RAVE Diet, stick to the proportions shown in the pyramid because this diet is satisfying and you'll consume a wide variety of foods eating this way. Your diet will evolve as you learn more about whole plant foods and you can change the proportions according to your preferences and dietary goals.

If you're concerned about an imbalance between Omega-3's and Omega-6's, follow the phrase "more greens, less grains," meaning you should make low-fat green vegetables the predominant part of your diet. If you want extra Omega-3, sprinkle some ground flaxseed on your food. (For more on the benefits of flaxseed, see *Essential Tips & Tricks*.)

Spices, herbs and sauces are throughout the pyramid. Use these to give your food added flavor. Spices and herbs, in particular, are calorie-free, rich in cancer-fighting nutrients and can turn plain-tasting foods into fabulous foods. (See *Rules for Meal Preparation – Flavorings*.) If you're not familiar with spices, you can start with Italian Seasoning, as that is universally liked, and branch out from there. If you think eating a plant-based diet is boring, you'll be pleasantly surprised once you learn how to use spices.

Organic foods are at the base of the pyramid. You should buy certified organic products whenever possible. These foods are grown without the use of chemical fertilizers and pesticides. Pesticides, in fact, reduce the amount of antioxidants in plants, so organic foods have higher cancer-fighting nutrients than conventionally grown foods. The reason for this is that plants use their own antioxidants in an effort to defend themselves against pesticides, thus lowering the antioxidants available to consumers.[1] (For more on organic foods, see *Reading Labels & Ingredients*.)

It's a lot easier than you think to follow the RAVE Diet. All you have to do is choose your favorite foods from the pyramid, follow the proportions – and Bingo! – you're doin' the RAVE. It's really as simple as that. Remember, plant foods are medicines. The more you eat, the healthier you're going to be.

For meal preparation guidelines, see *Rules for Meal Preparation*. And if you ever get stumped about what to eat, see *Food Lists*, which shows a sampling of just how many foods are available with the RAVE Diet.

Some people like to have meal plans, i.e., what to eat for the next two weeks, for example. I personally don't like them because what do you do after two weeks? If you want a meal plan, it's very simple to put together. Just select a recipe for breakfast, lunch and dinner for the next two weeks. You can select them at random, in sequence, or repeat the same ones. It's that easy.

Here are a few simple examples of the pyramid:

Breakfast
    Condiments
    Nuts
    Unsweetened juice/smoothie
    Fruits
    Oatmeal & breads

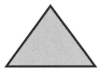

Lunch (salad)
    Seasonings/sauces
    Avocado
    Beans
    Low-fat vegetables
    Green leafy salad vegetables

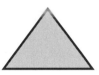

Dinner
    Seasonings/sauces
    Beans/peas
    Low-fat vegetables
    Rice/potatoes/bulgur, etc.

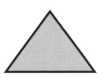

There are an infinite number of variations and, in this sense, there are no rules. You can tailor the diet to meet your specific tastes and dietary goals. Use the *Mix-Ins/Side Dishes* recipes to mix in your favorite foods with filler foods. The sample recipes contained in this book are just that – samples – because you will

---

[1] American Chemical Society Press Release, 3/3/03, printed in Journal of Agricultural and Food Chemistry, 2/26/03.

discover what you like and how you like to prepare your food on your own. Don't be afraid to substitute recipe ingredients, add vegetables to recipes or change them around. Everyone has their favorite plant foods and you will be able to fit them into the rules very simply. And don't worry about making a mistake. Too much ginger in a recipe, for example, can be easily covered up by adding other spices.

Reading Labels & Ingredients

Due to food industry lobbying designed to hide bad ingredients and confuse the customer, you almost have to attend night school to understand food labeling. Let's simplify it.

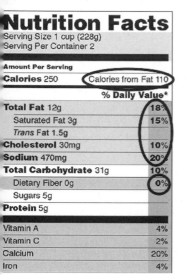

The label to the left is for macaroni and cheese (which you should never eat!). There are three circles you should focus on. The first is "Calories from Fat." Manufacturers rarely do the math for you, but this is 44 percent fat (110 / 250 = .44). Put it back on the shelf. You should ideally find products with zero fat or less than 10 percent fat.

Next are Total Fat, Saturated Fat and Cholesterol, shown as a percent of daily calories. Again, look for zeroes. You will find many choices of packaged products with these numbers at health food stores.

After cholesterol is sodium. This is a big item in packaged products because it's used as a preservative and percentages will vary all over the place. The lower, the better.

Look closely at the serving size because the trend is to make serving sizes smaller in order to disguise just how bad a product really is. Many candy bars, for example, are now two servings!

The last circle is Dietary Fiber, which is of great importance. In this case, the larger the number, the better.

A Simple Rule of Thumb About Fat

If you are trying to maintain a diet at 10 percent fat (which reverses heart disease), anything more than 1 gram of fat per 100 calories is higher than you want. If you are trying to prevent heart disease and do not have any risk factors, then 2 grams of fat per 100 calories is your maximum for a 20 percent fat diet.

Due to food industry lobbying, a product can be labeled "fat free" and it can list zero grams of fat, if the fat content is less than 0.5 grams of fat. This is how foods can have oil or high-fat ingredients listed in their Nutrition Facts label, yet contain "zero" fat. Fat free means less than 0.5 grams of fat per serving. Low fat means less than 3 grams of fat per serving.

When food manufacturers moved to fat free packaged goods, what they did in many products was add more sugar and simple (refined) carbohydrates to replace the fat, so instead of *eating* fat, you're quickly *creating* fat inside your body.

Ingredients

On ingredients lists, the top three ingredients to look for are:

Whole, sprouted wheat or organic rolled oats should be the first ingredient in any grain product, such as bread or cereal.

Hydrogenated oils: never purchase a product that contains the word "hydrogenated" anywhere in the ingredients.

Sugar, high fructose or fructose, sucrose, glucose, or sorbitol should never be the first, second or third ingredient. In fact, the best products have none of these ingredients.

Also, never purchase anything with the word "instant" on it, such as instant oatmeal.

There will also be a list of ingredients on the package with names most of us could never pronounce. Here is a *short* list of ingredients you should avoid:

all oils, especially hydrogenated oils (partially, fully or whatever)	lactic acid
	lactose
alum (as in aluminum)	lactulose
artificial colorings (any food dye)	lard
BHT	monodiglycerides
calcium propionate	monoglycerides
carrageenan (some are sensitive to this)	monosodium glutamate (MSG)
caseinogen	mycoprotein
casein	palmitate
collagen	polysorbates
diglycerides and monoglycerides	rennet
EDTA	rennin
gelatin	sodium caseinate
glycerin/glycerides	sodium nitrite
hydrolyzed vegetable protein	sugar (any form of sugar)
hydrolyzed oat flour	sulfites
hydrolyzed plant protein	vegetable oils, especially hydrogenated
hydrolysates	oils (partially, fully or whatever)
hydrogenated vegetable oils	whey

A comprehensive list of ingredients would require a book, so in general, if you can't pronounce it, don't put it in your mouth.[1] When in doubt, your best bet is to put the product back on the shelf and go for natural products that come in their natural packages.

Sticky Labels on Fruit

Ever noticed those little "brand" stickers on fruit? They tell you how the product was grown or "created."

There's a number on the label known as the "price look up" or PLU code that speeds up the check out process. But there's more to the PLU than just price.

Conventionally grown produce has a 4-number PLU code.

Genetically engineered produce has a 5-number PLU, beginning with 8.

Organically grown fruit has a 5-number PLU, beginning with 9.

Using this system for an apple, the numbering would look like this:

4011 - conventional grown apple
84011 - genetically engineered apple
94011 - organically grown apple

Organic Labeling

100 Percent Organic: Must contain only organically produced ingredients.

Organic: Defined by the USDA as containing 95 percent of organic ingredients.

Made With Organic: Must contain at least 70 percent organic ingredients. These foods cannot bear the USDA organic seal.

Some Organic Ingredients: Products with less than 70 percent organic ingredients are only allowed to list the organic items in the ingredient panel on the side of the package. These also cannot display the USDA organic seal.

Don't confuse the label "organic" with the label "natural." Natural is a loose term generally meaning that no artificial ingredients were added in processing and has nothing to do with how the product was grown or raised.

---

[1] The latest problem on this front involved "nano food additives," which utilize nanotechnology. Nanotechnology involves the design and manipulation of materials on molecular scales, smaller than the width of a human hair and invisible to the naked eye. These are being introduced into foods without any regulation, at the time of this writing, and people are rightly concerned about their safety. Using nanotechnologies in food is estimated to be a $20 billion market by 2010. Again, the best way to avoid such additives is to purchase whole, organic foods.

What Organic Means

Organic standards require that the land used to grow organic food go through a three year "transition period" to make sure the crops are free of synthetic pesticides and synthetic fertilizers.

All organic agriculture prohibits the use of synthetic pesticides and fertilizers, irradiation and sewage sludge. In addition, no genetically modified organisms can be contained in anything labeled organic.

Organic standards specify that animals may only be fed plant diets, with no animal by-products, which eliminates the risk of certain diseases, such as mad cow disease.

Organic products are also likely to taste better and be free of artificial preservatives and chemicals.

Rules for Meal Preparation

Cooking Without Oil

When sautéing, use about twice as much oil substitute (see below) as you would oil and add more oil substitute as necessary. This will vary, depending on what you are sautéing, but with a little experience you will get the hang of it. And remember, you can always add more oil substitute if needed. You'll soon discover you don't need even a drop of oil to make your food delicious – and it won't have that greasy taste, but the nice, natural taste of whole foods.

Cook on low or medium heat to avoid the oil substitute from evaporating too quickly. This will take a little longer than a high-heat oil-based sauté, but it's worth the wait because you're not sending the oil to your hips – or waist – and the food tastes so much cleaner! If you need to brown something, just turn up the heat to high at the end of the cooking, stir the food, and the water will oil substitute will evaporate quickly. Believe it or not, you can make delicious browned home fries using just water! The following are oil substitutes for sautéing and baking:

Oil Substitutes for

> **Sautéing:** water, apple juice, sherry, vegetable stock, wine, vinegars

> **Baking:** any pureed fruit, e.g., applesauce, apple butter, pureed bananas, pureed prunes

With baked goods, use the same amount of substitute, as you would oil. Many use baby food purees as a convenient substitute. Baby food purees work best if the puree is diluted with a little water.

Pressure Cooker Note: If you use a pressure cooker, many recipes call for added oil to prevent foaming, particularly for beans. You can eliminate the oil by putting a strip of kombu (dried seaweed available at health food stores), which will eliminate the foaming. Just remember to remove the kombu before you serve the dish. Newer pressure cookers do not have a problem with foaming.

Making Plain Foods Taste Fabulous

To most people, natural whole foods taste rather "plain," at least until your taste buds adjust and you come to enjoy the wide varieties of tastes inherent in whole, natural foods. The easiest and most delicious way to make these foods more exciting is to add seasonings and sauces.

I'm often asked, "How do you liven up your food?" It's easy with seasonings and sauces because there are hundreds you can choose from. What follows is a short list to get you started. The flavors of most whole plant foods are very subtle and they will easily take on whatever seasonings or sauces you care to use. Just be careful with commercial seasonings or custom mixes to make sure there is no added salt in them. You should avoid all salt seasonings, except for salt substitutes, such as Mrs. Dash or Salt Free Spike.

And don't be shy when you're dining out. If you eat a food that tastes delicious, ask the chef what seasonings he used with it.

Here is a short list of some of my favorite commercial seasonings:

Coriander
Cumin
Curry
Fajita Seasoning
Hungarian Hot Paprika
Italian Seasoning
Mint
Mustard
Oregano Leaf

Flavorings

The following lists various foods and the seasonings that are typically used with them. We then give a short list of seasonings, sauces, salad dressings, condiments and sweeteners. Of course, if you have a favorite seasoning, it can go with practically anything – because it's *your* favorite.

Seasonings, Sauces, Salad Dressings, Condiments & Sweeteners

Seasonings

Beans
Avocado, cayenne, chili, cumin, epazote, Mexican oregano, parsley, pepper, savory, sage, thyme
Breads
Anise, basil, cardamom, cinnamon, coriander, cumin, dill, garlic, lemon peel, orange peel, poppy, seeds, saffron, thyme, rosemary
Fruits
Anise, black pepper, cardamom, cinnamon, coriander, cumin, ginger, mint
Potatoes, rice
Basil, coriander, dill, oregano, paprika, parsley, poppy seeds, rosemary, thyme
Salads & Dressings
Basil, caraway, celery seed, fennel, garlic, ginger, lemon peel, mint, mustard, oregano, paprika, parsley, rosemary, thyme
Soups
Basil, bay, black pepper, chives, chili, cilantro, cumin, dill, fennel, garlic, paprika, parsley, rosemary, thyme
Sweets
Anise, cardamom, cinnamon, cloves, fennel, ginger, lemon peel, nutmeg, orange peel, rosemary, saffron
Vegetables
Chili, cumin, mustard, curry powder, garam masala, ginger, dill, cilantro, black pepper, garlic, mint, paprika, thyme, turmeric

Here is a description of some of the more common spices and their typical uses.

Allspice: Pungent, spicy, like a mix of nutmeg, cloves and cinnamon. Virtually anything, from salads to desserts.
Anise: Sweet, similar to licorice. Flavoring in cookies, candies and pastries.
Basil: Pungent, somewhat sweet. Tomato dishes, salads, cooked vegetables.
Bay leaves: Bitter, pungent. Soups, stews, tomato sauces. Remove leaf before serving
Black pepper: Pungent, somewhat hot. Virtually anything.
Borage: Mild. Garnish or in salads or in herbal tea mixtures.
Capers: Pungent. In sauces, as a garnish.
Caraway seeds: Sweet, nutty. Cookies and cakes, apple sauce, vinegars.
Cardamom: Sweet, pungent, fragrant, strong taste. Stews, curries.
Cayenne pepper: Very hot. In anything you want to taste hot.

Celery seed: Pungent celery flavor. Flavoring in tomato juice, sauces and soups.

Chervil: Similar to parsley. Flavoring in soups, casseroles, salads.

Chile powder: Spicy, hot. In chili or other spicy dishes.

Chives: Sharp, onion or garlic flavor. Fresh; frozen if fresh not available Garnish, added to salads.

Cilantro: Spicy, sweet or hot. Common ingredient in Mexican salsas.

Cinnamon: Sweet, fragrant. Sweet dishes, curries and stews.

Cloves: Sweet or bittersweet. Sweet dishes or as a contrast in stews and curries.

Coriander: Warm, aromatic. Cakes, cookies, breads, curries.

Cumin: Peppery, aromatic. Soups, stews, sauces.

Curry powder: Hot. Curries.

Dill: Bittersweet, cool. Potatoes, meats, breads, salads, sauces, curries.

Fennel: Similar to anise, but sweeter, lighter, warm. Salads, soups, stews.

Fenugreek: Sweet, somewhat like burnt sugar. Pastries, beverages, syrups.

Garlic: Pungent, onion-like. Roasted, or flavoring for pasta sauces. Good in any dish meal.

Ginger: Mix of pepper and sweetness. Cakes, breads, cookies, Asian dishes.

Green peppercorns: Mild, slightly sweet. Vinegars, in sauces.

Horseradish: Sharp, similar to mustard. As condiment.

Lovage: Similar to celery, but stronger. Use as you would celery, in soups, stews, salads.

Mace: Similar to nutmeg, but stronger. Custards, spice cakes, fruit desserts.

Marjoram: Delicate taste. Soups, stews, marinades.

Mint: Sweet, aromatic, cooling. Salads, vegetables.

Mustard, brown: Sharp, pungent, hotter than yellow mustard. Use as condiment.

Mustard, yellow: Hot, tangy, less of a bite than brown mustard. Use as a condiment.

Nutmeg: Warm, spicy, sweet. Cakes, cookies, sweet potatoes.

Oregano: Delicate taste. Pasta dishes, chili, vegetables, soups.

Paprika: Sweet, warm. Soups, potato salad.

Parsley: Mildly peppery. Garnish in sauces, soups and salads.

Poppy seed: Nutty, aromatic. Muffins, cakes, salad dressings.

Rosemary: Aromatic. Sauces, vegetables.

Saffron: Pungent, aromatic, fragrant. Rice, stews, curries.

Sage: Musty, slightly bitter. Stews, vegetables.

Sesame seed: Nutty. Breads, salad dressings.

Star Anise: Very similar to anise. Flavoring in cookies, candies and pastries.

Summer savory: Cross between thyme and mint, milder than winter savory. Soups, bean dishes.

Tarragon: Sweet, pungent. Vegetables.

Thyme: Minty, lemony. Soups, salads, cooked vegetables.

Turmeric: Pungent, somewhat bitter, warm. Curries. Primary ingredient in yellow commercial mustard.
Vanilla: Sweet, aromatic, fragrant. Desserts.
White pepper: Similar to black peppercorn, milder. As a condiment.
Winter savory: Combination of thyme and mint. Soups, bean dishes, vegetables.

Sauces

You can, of course, make your own sauces, but there are hundreds of commercial brands that are available and more convenient to use. Experiment and mix your favorite sauces together to create a new sauce just for you. Here are just a few of my favorites:

A1 Steak sauce
Barbeque sauce
Black bean sauce
Chipotle sauce
Cranberry sauce
Dijon Mustard
Hoisin sauce
Hot pepper sauce
Plum sauce
Salsa
Tamari (soy sauce - low-sodium, or Bragg Liquid Aminos if sensitive to soy)
Tabasco sauce
Teriyaki sauce (low-sodium)
Tomato sauce
Tomato ketchup
Vegetarian Worcestershire sauce

Note: Ingredients will vary for a particular sauce, depending on who makes it, so inspect the label closely before purchasing it.

A Better Tomato Sauce

Very few prepared pasta sauces do not contain oil and are low in sodium. The best way is to simply make your own – and it's incredibly easy.

All you have to do is purchase cans (or jars) of tomato sauce and canned or fresh cut tomatoes. (Note: there should not be oil or sodium added).

Just chop up some of your favorite vegetables (or throw them in a food processor), mix them into the tomato sauce with the tomatoes and add your favorite herbs or just use Italian seasoning and Voila! You have your own pasta sauce.

You can flavor the sauce however you want. I usually add some Tabasco sauce or horseradish to give it a little zing. Or feel free to add any other spices, herbs or sauces for flavor. Once you get it down, you'll have a pasta sauce that tastes the way you like it. As you'll discover, the taste is much cleaner than the oily stuff sold on the shelf.

If you like it fresher (I do), here is a simple way to make your own tomato sauce from scratch.

Easy Tomato Sauce

6 Roma tomatoes, coarsely chopped
1 clove garlic, minced
1 or 2 sprigs fresh basil leaves
1/4 teaspoon ground black pepper

Combine all the ingredients in the food processor and process to a smooth or chunky sauce, as desired.

Salad Dressings Without Oil

Balsamic vinaigrette dressings
Other vinegar-based dressings
Salad dressings (oil-free)

Cuisine Perel makes a wide range of vinegar-based dressings that are fabulous. www.gourmetofoldecity.com/perelvinegars.html

Make Your Own[2]

These are quick and simple recipes to make delicious oil-free salad dressings. Simply increase the proportions to make larger amounts. The directions are the same for all dressings: simply combine all ingredients.

---

[2] Some of these recipes were adapted from Mary Clifford, RD , Flavorful Salad Dressings Without the Oil!, Vegetarian Journal May/June 1999 and CancerProject.org.

Balsamic Vinaigrette

1/3 cup balsamic vinegar
1/4 cup apple cider vinegar
1 tbsp water
2 tsp mustard

Blackstrap-Mustard Vinaigrette

1/4 cup apple-cider vinegar
4-5 tsp blackstrap molasses (unsulfured)
1 tsp mustard

Garlicky-Tomato Dressing

1 garlic clove pressed
1/4 cup vegetable juice
1 tsp lemon juice
1/4 tsp Italian seasoning

Italian Dressing

1/4 cup red-wine vinegar
1 tbsp lemon juice
1/2 tsp dried minced onion
1/4 tsp oregano
1/4 tsp basil
Pinch of thyme
Pinch of garlic powder

Mustard/Balsamic Vinaigrette

1/3 cup balsamic vinegar
1/3 cup mustard of choice
1/4 cup apple cider vinegar
1 tsp water

Mustard/Garlic Vinaigrette #1

½ cup rice vinegar
2 tsp mustard
1 garlic clove pressed

Mustard/Garlic Vinaigrette #2
Makes 3-4 cups

2-3 medium garlic cloves
1/2 cup mustard
3 tbsp lemon juice or rice or cider vinegar
3 tbsp water
1 tsp light miso
1 tsp low-sodium Tamari (soy sauce)
1/2 tsp maple syrup
1/2 tsp curry powder

Raspberry Vinaigrette

1 clove garlic
3/4 cup water
1/4 cup raspberry vinegar
1/2 inch sliced shallot
2 tbsp walnuts
1 tsp Dijon mustard
1/4 tsp basil

Tomato Vinaigrette

1 clove garlic pressed
¾ cup tomato juice
3 tbsp apple vinegar
1 tbsp lemon juice
1 tsp mustard

Condiments

Applesauce
Banana chips
Cilantro
Corn relishes
Ginger
Hummus
Lemon juice
Lime juice

Mustards
Mushrooms
Olives
Pickles
Potatoes
Salsa
Sunflower seeds
Tomato sauce

Sweeteners

All of the sweeteners listed below, although healthier than refined sugar, should be used very sparingly, if at all. Ideally, only fresh or dried whole fruits should be used as sweeteners.

Agave nectar	Maple sugar
Barley malt syrup	Maple syrup
Brown rice syrup	Molasses (black strap)
Concentrated fruit juice syrups	Organic unrefined cane sugar.
Date sugar (ground, dehydrated dates)	Organic dairy-free chocolate
	Sorghum syrup
Fresh or dried fruits	Turbinado sugar

Bean Preparation

Beans are an excellent source of nutrients. Although they tend to be high in fat, they should be eaten occasionally. The most convenient way to eat beans is right from the can, but in the can they are high in sodium and other preservatives, so it is best to avoid that.

Purchasing dry beans in bulk is much healthier (sodium free, preservative free and process free), they are cheaper than canned beans and they are more environmentally friendly (less energy expended in production, less energy expended in recycling and less material used for packaging). And with a little planning, dry beans can be prepped and cooked very easily.

First, always rinse dry beans using a colander and pick out any defective or broken beans or debris, such as twigs, etc.

Next you must soak them. Soaking helps break down the complex sugars (oligosaccharides) in beans, which will greatly reduce or eliminate flatulence. A soaked bean is more likely to retain its maximum nutritional value.

When soaking, beans will rehydrate to at least twice their dry size, so be sure to start with a large enough pot and use about twice the amount of water as beans. How can you tell if a bean is fully soaked? Cut a bean open. If the bean is undersoaked, you'll notice the core is chalky, as if a kernel of rice was in the center. If the bean is fully soaked, it has an even color all the way through.

Quick Soak: Bring a pot of water to boil, add the dry beans and let them boil for about two to three minutes. After boiling, turn off the heat, cover and let them soak in the hot water for one to two hours. After you have soaked them, drain the beans, add fresh water (approx an inch above the beans) and cook until tender.

Long Soak: Put the dry beans in a large bowl or pot of room temperature water (too cold or hot will affect the beans negatively). Add water. Let them sit for 8 to 10 hours, or overnight. After soaking, drain the beans and add fresh water (approx an inch above the beans). Bring to a boil, then reduce the heat and cook until tender. Add seasonings to taste during cook time, if desired.

Cooking times will vary, depending on the bean, but will generally range from 45 minute to an hour and a half. The big exception is soy beans, which can take three to four hours to cook.

Pressure Cooking: When using a pressure cooker, you can either soak the beans or eliminate that step altogether. We recommend soaking because it still helps break down the complex sugars. Either way, put the beans in the pressure cooker, adding three times as much water as beans. Cook at 15 pounds of pressure for 30 minutes for small beans. For large beans, such as limas or fava beans, pressure cook for about 40 minutes. Note: if you have an old pressure cooker, you can eliminate foaming by putting in a strip of kombu (dried seaweed available at health food stores). Newer pressure cookers do not have a problem with foaming.

Fresh Beans:[1] Fresh beans are not as readily available as dry beans, but they can be found in farmer's markets. You will have to first shell the beans before cooking.

There are two basic methods of cooking fresh beans: boiling or steaming. To boil, drop the shelled beans into boiling water and cover. Boil gently for five to ten minutes. To steam, put about an inch of water into the bottom of a saucepan, and then place the beans into a steamer basket (that will fit into the saucepan). Cover the pan and steam over boiling water for five to ten minutes.

Note: after fresh fava beans are cooked, their tough skins are usually peeled and discarded. When left on, they give the beans a bitter flavor. To peel the skins, us a small paring knife and peel away one end. Then squeeze the opposite end and the bean will slip out easily.

Microwaves

Some 90 percent of modern households have microwave ovens and there is a lot of controversy about their safety and what they do to food. You will find countless articles on the internet claiming that microwaving is unsafe. Most of these claims are unsubstantiated. For example, there is the case of Norma Levitt who was given a blood transfusion with blood heated in a microwave oven and died shortly thereafter. People cite this as "proof" the microwave "somehow" altered Ms. Levitt's blood and that was what killed her. In fact, a jury found that Norman Levitt died of a blood clot, not of microwaved blood.[2]

---

[1] This preparation advice is from Zel and Reuben Allen, Vegetarians in Paradise.
[2] www.wyom.state.wy.us/applications/oscn/deliverdocument.asp?citeid=4387 This is the reference to the civil case regarding Norma Levitt. Microwaving blood is never a good idea in the first place. Heating blood with a microwave destroys red blood cells, which

Surprisingly, there have not been comprehensive studies on the effect of microwave cooking with respect to human health, so we do not have a good basis for judging health concerns in this regard. Despite this and the fact that people have reversed cancers while microwaving their food, I would recommend you *not* use microwaves at all. Despite the fact there is not conclusive evidence microwaves are unsafe, there *is* some evidence they are, so to be on the safe side, I recommend against them. Microwaving is a convenience, not a necessity, so it can easily be discontinued.

In one very small study,[3] it was found that microwaved food produced changes in the subjects' blood and immune function. These included a decrease in hemoglobin, an increase in hemotocrit and leukocytes and a decrease in lymphocytes. There was also an increase in the activity of certain bacteria in the food as well as the appearance of altered cells resembling the pathogenic stages that occur in the early development of some cancers. In the food itself, there was increased acidity, damaged protein molecules, enlarged fat cells and decreased amounts of folic acid.

Collecting, freezing and reheating breast milk is standard practice in most neonatal units in the US. In a study by Stanford University School of Medicine, it was found that human breast milk loses some of its abilities to fight infection when reheated with a microwave oven. It also weakened antibodies and proteins that inhibit bacterial growth and help infants ward off infection.[4]

Chemicals used in "microwave safe" packaging, such as found in microwave popcorn, pizza, etc. can migrate into food.[5] The FDA has been made aware of this, but they have failed to regulate the problem.

There are also claims that nutrients are lost when microwaving food. This is not supported by scientific evidence. The reality is that *every* cooking method can destroy vitamins and other nutrients in food. The factors that determine the extent of destruction are how long the food is cooked, how much liquid is used and the cooking temperature, not whether the food was microwaved.

For example, a recent study[6] showed that microwaving broccoli removed anywhere from 74 to 97 percent of flavonoids, a vital nutrient that fights not just

---

can result in "gross hemolysis" of the blood, releasing large amounts of potassium. Excessive potassium, when introduced into the body, can be fatal. This was not the case with Norma Levitt, however.

[3] Bernard H. Blanc and Hans U. Hertel, "Influence on Man: Comparative Study About Food Prepared Conventionally and in the Microwave Oven," Raum & Zeit, 3(2): 1992.

[4] Quan R, et al., Effects of microwave radiation on anti-infective factors in human milk, Pediatrics. 1992 Apr;89(4 Pt 1):667-9; Microwaving Breast Milk, Microwave News, May/June 1992, p. 14. See also, G. Lubec et al., Aminoacid Isomerisation and Microwave Exposure, Lancet 2(8676):1392-93, 1989.

[5] David Steinman and Samuel S. Epstein, M.D., Safe Shopper's Bible (New York: Macmillan, 1995).

cancer, but cardiovascular and other diseases. However, the nutrients were not "lost," but were leached out of the vegetable into the water that was used for cooking. If you include the water with your meal, you have theoretically not lost any nutrients at all. In comparison, boiling broccoli removed 66 percent of the flavonoids and pressure cooking leached out 47 percent. Quick and simple steaming was the best method and had only minimal losses. The loss of micronutrients by any cooking method is one reason I recommend at least half of your food be eaten uncooked. (See *Essential Dietary Guidelines*)

Environmental Exposure to Microwaves

While many are concerned about microwaving their food, they are also busy talking on their cell phones, computing over WiFi (wireless) connections and exposing themselves to microwaves in their own environment. The ambient radiation has increased dramatically over the last few decades and this can potentially be more dangerous than microwaving food.

Symptoms known to be caused by exposure to electromagnetic radiation – depending on frequency, duration, and exposure levels – range from decreased stamina, memory problems, fatigue, sleep disturbances, headaches, eye sensitivities, increased allergies and dizziness to insomnia, swollen lymph nodes, depression, loss of appetite, hypoxia (lack of oxygen getting to the tissues), vision problems, weakened immune system, frequent urination, night sweats and so on.[7] Not surprisingly, such symptoms often appear suddenly in people who have had a cell phone tower installed near their home.

---

[6] F Vallejo, FA Tomás-Barberán, C García-Viguera, Phenolic compound contents in edible parts of broccoli inflorescences after domestic cooking, Journal of the Science of Food and Agriculture, Volume 83 Issue 14 , Pages 1389 - 1538 (November 2003). See also, Fumio Watanabe, et al., Effects of Microwave Heating on the Loss of Vitamin B12 in Foods, J. Agric. Food Chem., 1998, 46 (1), pp 206–210.

[7] Becker, R.O., The Body Electric, pp. pp. 314-315; Cherry N. (1996). "Swiss shortwave transmitter study sounds warning." Electromagnetics Forum , Vol. 1, No. 2 Article 10; Microwave News. Sept/Oct. page 14; Kolodynski AA, Kolodynska VV. (1996). "Motor and psychological functions of school children living in the area of the Skrunda Radio Location Station in Latvia." Sci Total Environ. Feb 2;180(1):87-93; Santini R, Santini P, Danze JM, Le Ruz P, Seigne M. (2002). "Investigation on the health of people living near mobile telephone relay stations: I/Incidence according to distance and sex." Pathol Biol (Paris). [Article in French] Jul; 50(6):369-73; Al-Khlaiwi T, Meo SA. (2004). "Association of mobile phone radiation with fatigue, headache, dizziness, tension and sleep disturbance in Saudi population." Saudi Medical Journal, Jun; 25(6): 732-6; Bortkiewicz A, Zmyslony M, Szyjkowska A, Gadzicka E. (2004). "Subjective symptoms reported by people living in the vicinity of cellular phone." Med Pr.; 55 (4):345-51. See also Do You Have Microwave/EMR Sickness? by Paul Raymond Doyon. Much of this discussion and references is based on this article. It can be found on the internet by searching the title.

Studies on the effects of ambient radiation in microwave ovens, cell phones, cordless phones, fluorescent lighting, transformers, cell phone towers, electrical substations and power lines have shown that exposure can induce the following:

- An abnormal flux of calcium into and out of cells, which can trigger or aggravate allergic reactions.[8]
- An increase in allergies[9] due to an increase in the production of histamine, the chemical responsible for allergic reactions.[10]
- An increase in immunoglobulin antibodies in the body, which are responsible for triggering an allergic reaction to a particular substance or protein.[11]
- Mitochondria dysfunction, which is the powerhouse of human cells. This may cause fatigue as well as other problems.[12]

---

[8] Amara S, Abdelmelek H & Sakly M. (2004). "Effects of acute exposure to magnetic field ionic composition of frog sciatic nerve." Pakistani Journal of Medical Science. 20(2) 91-96; Cellphones - a boon to modern society or a threat to human health? An interview with Dr Neil Cherry, NZine (online), 6/01/03.

[9] Kimata H. (2003). Enhancement of allergic skin wheal responses in patients with atopic eczema/dermatitis syndrome by playing video games or by a frequently ringing mobile phone. Eur J Clin Invest. Jun: 33(6):513-7; Kimata H. (2005). Microwave radiation from cellular phones increases allergen-specific IgE production. Allergy. Jun;60(6):838-9; Kimata H. (2002). Enhancement of allergic skin wheal responses by microwave radiation from mobile phones in patients with atopic eczema/dermatitis syndrome. Int Arch Allergy Immunol. Dec;129(4):348-50.

[10] Johansson O, et al., Cutaneous mast cells are altered in normal healthy volunteers sitting in front of ordinary TVs/PCs--results from open-field provocation experiments. J Cutan Pathol. 2001 Nov;28(10):513-9; Johansson O, Hilliges M, Han SW. A screening of skin changes, with special emphasis on neurochemical marker antibody evaluation, in patients claiming to suffer from screen dermatitis as compared to normal healthy controls. Exp Dermatol (1996) 5: 279-285.

[11] Bergier L, Lisiewicz J, et al. Effect of electromagnetic radiation on T-lymphocyte subpopulations and immunoglobulin level in human blood serum after occupational exposure. Med Pr.;41(4):211-5 (1990); Dmoch A., Moszczynski P. (1998). Levels of immunoglobulin and subpopulations of T lymphocytes and NK cells in men occupationally exposed to microwave radiation in frequencies of 6-12 GHz. Med Pr. 49(1):45-9; Moszczynski P, Lisiewicz J, Dmoch A, Zabinski Z, Bergier L, Rucinska M, Sasiadek U. The effect of various occupational exposures to microwave radiation on the concentrations of immunoglobulins and T lymphocyte subsets. Wiad Lek. 52(1-2):30-4 (1999); Yuan ZQ, et al. Effect of low intensity and very high frequency electromagnetic radiation on occupationally exposed personnel. Zhonghua Lao Dong Wei Sheng Zhi Ye Bing Za Zhi. Aug: 22(4):267-9 (2004); Kimata H. Microwave radiation from cellular phones increases allergen-specific IgE production. Allergy. Jun;60(6):838-9 (2005).

[12] Gerald Goldberg, M.D., Would You Put Your Head in a Microwave Oven?, 2006; Buchachenko AL, et al. New mechanisms of biological effects of electromagnetic fields. Biofizika, May-Jun;51(3):545-52 (2006).

124 - The RAVE Diet & Lifestyle

- A decrease in the numbers of Natural Killer (NK) cells, the body's first line of defense against pathogens and extremely important when fighting cancer.[13]
- A weakened immune system.[14]
- An increase in viruses, bacteria, mold, parasites, and yeast in the blood of the human host.
- "Subliminal" stress (since the body does not know it is under stress), which causes the adrenal glands to excrete abnormally greater amounts of cortisol and adrenaline. This can lead to irritability and hyperactivity. If continued it could eventually lead to adrenal exhaustion, which is commonly found in chronic fatigue syndrome.[15]
- A decrease in levels of the brain hormone norepinephrine,[16] which is essential for control of the autonomic nervous system. If not working properly, the body will have trouble regulating its temperature.[17] People with chronic fatigue syndrome have been found to have a disturbed circadian core body temperature.[18] A decrease in norepinephrine levels has also been connected to short-term memory disturbances, ADHD and depression.
- Alteration of the production of the brain hormone melatonin, which is necessary for proper sleep.[19]

---

[13] Smialowicz RJ, Rogers RR, Garner RJ, Riddle MM, Luebke RW, Rowe DG. Microwaves (2,450 MHz) suppress murine natural killer cellactivity. Bioelectromagnetics. 4(4):371-81 (1983); Nakamura H, et al. Effects of exposure to microwaves on cellular immunity and placental steroids in pregnant rats. Occup Environ Med, Sep;54(9):676-80 (1997); Yang H.K., et al. Effects of microwave exposure on the hamster immune system. I. Natural killer cell activity. Bioelectromagnetics. 1983; 4(2): 123-39.

[14] Levitt, B. Blake, Electromagnetic Fields, pp. 128-129, 1995. See also, Immune system attacked by mobile phones, BBC News, October 15, 1998.

[15] Levitt BB. Electromagnetic Fields, 1995.

[16] Takahashi A, et al. Aspects of hypothalamic neuronal systems in VMH lesion-induced obese rats." Journal of Autonomic Nervous System. Aug;48(3):213-9 (1994).

[17] Gandhi VC, Ross DH. Alterations in alpha-adrenergic and muscarinic cholinergic receptor binding in rat brain following nonionizing radiation." Radiation Res. Jan; 109(1):90-9 (1987).

[18] Tomoda A, et al. Disturbed circadian core body temperature rhythm and sleep disturbance in school refusal children and adolescents." Biol Psychiatry. Apr 1; 41(7): 810-3 (1997).

[19] Altpeter E.S, et al. Effect of short-wave (6-22 MHz) magnetic fields on sleep quality and melatonin cycle in humans: the Schwarzenburg shut-down study. Bioelectromagnetics. Feb: 27(2):142-50 (2006).

- Changes the level of the brain hormone, dopamine (or dopamine transporters), which has been linked with depression and restless leg syndrom.[20]
- An abnormal drop in the levels of the neurotransmitter acetylcholine, which has been linked to a number of neurological and neuromuscular disorders.[21]
- Alterations in regional cerebral blood flow, which corresponds to altered blood flow in conditions such as chronic fatigue syndrome.[22]

In addition to the above, recent studies have found links between cell phone use and the development of brain tumors and other cancers.[23] One these studies found that your risk of developing a brain tumor is 240 percent higher if you spend an hour a day on your cell over several years, versus someone who never used one.

Of course, all these studies show "links" and not conclusive proof or causation. On the opposite end of the spectrum, there have also been studies[24] in which mammary-tumor-prone animals were exposed to chronic, long-term microwave bandwidths and there were no differences between the exposed

---

[20] Brown AS, Gershon S. Dopamine and depression. J Neural Transm Gen . Sect. 91(2-3): 75-109 (1993); Allen R. Dopamine and iron in the pathophysiology of restless legs syndrome (RLS). Sleep Medicine, Jul;5(4):385-91 (2004).

[21] Omura Y, Losco M. Electro-magnetic fields in the home environment (color TV, computer monitor, microwave oven, cellular phone, etc) as potential contributing factors for the induction of oncogen C-fos Ab1, oncogen C-fos Ab2, integrin alpha 5 beta 1 and development of cancer, as well as effects of microwave on amino acid composition of food and living human brain." Acupunct Electrother Res. Jan-Mar;18(1):33-73 (1993); Testylier G, et al. Effects of exposure to low level radiofrequency fields on acetylcholine release in hippocampus of freely moving rats. Bioelectromagnetics. May: 23(4):249-55 (2002).

[22] Aalto S, Haarala C, et al. Mobile phone affects cerebral blood flow in humans. Journal of Cerebral Blood Flow Metab. Jul; 26(7):885-90 (2006); Huber R, et al. Exposure to pulse-modulated radio frequency electromagnetic fields affects regional cerebral blood flow. European Journal of Neuroscience, Feb; 21(4):1000-6 (2005).

[23] Lennart Hardell, et al. Pooled analysis of two case–control studies on use of cellular and cordless telephones and the risk for malignant brain tumours diagnosed in 1997–2003. Volume 79, Number 8 / September, 2006; Ken K. Karipidis, et al. Occupational exposure to ionizing and non-ionizing radiation and risk of non-Hodgkin lymphoma. Volume 80, Number 8 / August, 2007. See also Extensive Cell Phone Use Linked To Brain Tumors, Swedish Study, Medical News Today, April 1, 2006 www.medicalnewstoday.com/articles/40764.php.

[24] Frei MR, et al., Chronic exposure of cancer-prone mice to low-level 2450 MHz radiofrequency radiation, Bioelectromagnetics. 1998;19(1):20-31; Frei MR, et al., Chronic, low-level (1.0 W/kg) exposure of mice prone to mammary cancer to 2450 MHz microwaves, Radiat Res. 1998 Nov;150(5):568-76.

animals and the control animals. Other studies[25] have exposed animal fetus' to microwave radiation to see if it affected their brain development and it did not.

The bottom line is that there are conflicting studies out there, and the controversy over microwaves will continue.

There are, no doubt, individuals who may be more sensitive to electromagnetic fields and/or radiation than others may be. There are no tests for this sensitivity, but if you move out of a highly charged environment, the symptoms do go away quickly and you should notice a difference within a day.

In the interest of lowering your toxic burden, I would suggest you eliminate your microwave oven, since it's only a convenience (get a Turbo Oven), and minimize your use of a cell phone and any other appliance that may emit radiation. You should also use wired connections for your computer and replace your CRT with a flat-panel monitor.

If you think you may be affected by microwaves, take a vacation, leave your cell phone at home – and live a little!

Fast Food: Meals in Minutes

Most of us come home from work and the last thing we want to do is cook a meal. For myself, I usually open the refrigerator or pantry door and see what I have on-hand, then prepare a quick meal.

If this is you, one of the best ways to eat is to open your freezer door and "pour" out a meal using frozen vegetables. Frozen fruits and vegetables are almost as good as fresh and sometimes better (in terms of nutrients) because they're often picked and processed at their peak of ripeness, using techniques that lock in a slew of nutrients. They're also better than canned because most don't have added sodium. Any grocery store will have bags of frozen vegetables you can use.

Just pour them into a bowl, stir-fry them together. Add spices or stir in some tomato sauce with spices and Voila! You have a meal in minutes.

What about work? Again, think frozen. Just pour some vegetables into a container and take it to work. By lunchtime, the vegetables are pretty much thawed. Heat it up and you have lunch. Of course, if the only heating apparatus is a microwave, then think along the lines of a salad or other uncooked fruits and vegetable mixes.

I sometimes make a large pot of rice every week. Use any "filler" food like rice or potatoes as the base and pour frozen vegetables into it. Add tomato or another sauce, stir it up and you have your meal in minutes.

---

[25] Dr. Minoru Inouye, et al., Effect of 2,450 MHz microwave radiation on the development of the rat brain, Teratology, vol. 28, no. 3, pp. 413-419.

If you're on the go and like fast meals, you should set aside some time on the weekend to cook large amounts of food, then refrigerate or freeze it in serving sizes appropriate for your appetite. The idea is not that you eat the same meal seven days in a row, but that you build a supply of various meals. This will work like magic and you'll spend far less time preparing large meals suitable for re-heating, than you would preparing separate, individual meals.

Here are a few samples. It's not the foods used below, as much as the technique because you can substitute any foods for a quick meal, depending on what you have in the refrigerator or pantry.

3-Step Quickie

1) Cut up assorted vegetables and sauté or stir-fry them in water or a vegetable broth. Cook over medium heat.

2) Stir in your favorite seasonings and sauce (e.g., tomato sauce, black bean sauce, curry, Thai sauce, etc. See *Seasonings* and *Sauces*).

3) Serve on a bed of your favorite "filler" food, like brown rice or potatoes.

Rice, Beans & Vegetables

Brown rice in the bottom of the bowl (rice usually prepared beforehand in large quantities).

When finished, add cut raw or steamed vegetables and beans.

Mix-in any tomato or other sauce for flavoring, along with herbs and spices and heat it in a pan.

Any and All Vegetable Soup

Cut up your favorite vegetables in large quantities. Put them all in a pot full of water (large enough to handle your vegetables).

Add your favorite herbs, spices and sauces.

Cook until done. (Note that crock-pots or pressure cookers are ideal for this.)

This will last for days or longer and can be stored in the refrigerator or freezer.

When ready to eat, just heat it up and serve.

Keeping Brown Rice

I usually prepare a large quantity of brown rice using a rice cooker. This is a great investment because it takes me literally two minutes to prepare the rice and when it's done, the cooker goes into automatic warmer mode so I don't have to watch over it.

Just add the brown rice and twice the amount of water, e.g., 1 cup rice = 2 cups water.

Add seasonings to taste.

Press the appropriate buttons and you're done.

Rice can be stored in the refrigerator. It will cake and stick together, but will be fine once you heat it up again in a small amount of water.

Transition Foods

You can continue to enjoy many of your favorite meals by using substitutes, so don't throw away your existing cookbooks just yet. You can adapt your recipes easily or just make the "side dishes" in your traditional cookbook, the main dishes.

There are all kinds of meat and dairy substitutes available at supermarkets, and a much wider selection at health food stores. Don't be shy about asking about a substitute at your grocery or health food store. These substitutes can be used initially as a bridge to a 100 percent RAVE Diet – or as an occasional treat. Their biggest benefit is they contain no cholesterol and they are generally lower in fat. But like all packaged goods, they usually have high levels of sodium. Most of these products are made from soy, which is high in fat, so go easy on them. Inspect the fat content and ingredients label closely. (See *Reading Labels & Ingredients*.)

Some people get hooked on processed soy products like veggie burgers or dogs and think they're eating a plant-based diet – and wonder why they're not realizing the health benefits of this diet! Processed soy products are really "refined" foods and most of the nutrients have been lost in the refining process. Products such as seitan, tempeh, tofu, textured vegetable protein (TVP) and other refined soy (and rice) products should only be eaten as you transition to a natural, 100 percent plant-based RAVE Diet of unrefined plant foods.

Lastly, do not expect substitutes to taste like the original. Some are very close, but others will disappoint you. Our advice: don't attempt to continue your old eating habits with substitutes. The point of the RAVE Diet is to *change* your old eating habits, so use substitutes only as an occasional bridge to a new way of eating.

Meat, Dairy & Other Substitutes

Here's a short list of substitutes for common meat, dairy and other products. If you're not familiar with many of these products, just go to your health food store and ask for help.

Butter: butter substitutes
Buttermilk: clabbered soymilk (mix 2 teaspoons white vinegar or lemon juice per cup of soymilk)
Cheese: rice, soy or nut-based cheeses
Cottage cheese or ricotta: crumbled tofu
Cream Cheese: soy substitute
Eggs: psysillium seeds (mix with water), egg replacers, crumbled or pureed tofu
Gelatin: agar-agar, arrowroot, ground nuts and seeds, gums, kudzu
Gravies: soy substitutes

Half & Half: rice, soy substitute

Ice cream: soy/rice ice creams

Mayonnaise: soy mayonnaise

Meat, chicken or seafood stock: apple, cranberry, orange or pomegranate juice, garlic broth, miso (soybean paste) diluted with water, sherry, vegetable bouillon cubes, vegetable stock, wine, beer

Meat: potatoes, rice, beans, corn, cauliflower, seitan (from wheat), tempeh (from soy), textured vegetable protein, tofu. Everything from bacon to burgers to hot dogs, sausages, turkey and shrimp has a commercially available substitute – but go easy on them because they are refined products.

Meats, smoked: chipotle chilies, roasted vegetables, toasted nuts, smoked tofu

Milk: soymilk, nut milk, rice milk, oat milk

Oil for sautéing: apple juice, sherry, vegetable stock, wine; Balsamic vinegar

Oil in baked goods: any pureed fruit, e.g., applesauce, apple butter, pureed bananas, pureed prunes

Salad dressing: non-oil dressings, vinegar-based dressings, citrus juices

Salt: Mrs. Dash, Salt-Free Spike

Sausage: crumbled tofu seasoned with favorite spices

Sour Cream: soy sour cream

Sugar (refined): maple syrup, bananas, barley malt syrup, molasses, brown rice syrup, raw organic sugar, dried fruits, fruit juices

Whipped Cream: soy substitute

White flour (for baking): whole wheat flour, buckwheat flour, brown rice flour, oat flour, soy flour, barley, buckwheat, corn, kamut, oats, rice, rye, spelt

White sauce: pureed white beans

Yogurt: soy substitute

Recipes on the Web

The recipes contained in this book are meant to be only representative samples and a book cannot contain the wealth of possible meals that can be made with the RAVE Diet. To that end, there are thousands of recipes you can conveniently look up and search for on the Internet. Below are just a few of the web sites containing recipes for every occasion.

Just remember the rules when preparing recipes: substitute whole foods for refined foods (e.g., white pasta with whole wheat pasta) and use oil substitutes. (See *Cooking Without Oil*.)

The best and most extensive recipe archive, in my opinion, is the first one, FatFree.com.

FatFree.com
www.fatfree.com/
Asian Recipes
www.asiarecipe.com/
Healthy Heart Handbook Recipes
www.heart.kumu.org/
Recipe Source
www.recipesource.com/special-diets/vegetarian/
The Vegan Chef
www.veganchef.com/
Vegetarians in Paradise
www.vegparadise.com/recipeindex.html
VegWeb Recipes
www.vegweb.com/food/

Sample Recipes

The following presents a wide variety of recipes. If you wish to follow a "transition diet," you can substitute your favorite fruit juice or non-dairy milk instead of water as a moistener.

Breakfast Suggestions

Avocado slices on whole wheat bread
Baked apple with raisins and cinnamon
Mixed fruits (cantaloupe, banana, peaches, pears, apples, etc.)
Oatmeal with berries
Whole grain cereal with raisins, bananas, ground flaxseed
Flaxseed muffins
Fruit smoothie
Sliced bananas with raw carob powder sprinkled on top
Buckwheat, oat flour and flaxseed pancakes

Be your own chef. If you don't particularly like the texture of rolled oats, for example, mix-in Grape-Nuts with them and have your very own designer-breakfast the way you like it. Instead of using jellies and jams, try spreading whole fruits on toast, such as a pureed banana.

Anything "instant," such as instant oatmeal, should be put back on the shelf.

Cereals
Here are some of the more popular cereal brands, which contain whole grains. Be sure to inspect the ingredients list, as food manufacturers change ingredients over time. (See *Reading Labels & Ingredients*.)

Whole grains - Cold
Arrowhead Mills Organic Amaranth Flakes
Erewhon Crispy Brown Rice (like Rice Krispies)
Grape-Nuts (not flakes)
Health Valley Organic Fiber 7 Multigrain flakes
Heart-To-Heart (Kashi)
Nature's Path Organic Cereals
Puffed Wheat
Raisin Bran
Quaker Old-Fashioned (rolled) Oats (not instant)
Shredded wheat

Whole grains - Hot
Oat bran
Oatmeal (never buy instant oatmeal)
Quaker Multigrain
Quaker Old-Fashioned (rolled) Oats (not instant)
Ralston High Fiber
Roman Meal
Steel-cut Oats (the best oatmeal)
Wheatena

Fruit Drinks and Other Popular Breakfast Items

Most fruit drinks are bad for you and no more nutritious than carbonated soft drinks. The number one ingredient in most fruit drinks, including Gatorade, V8, Minute Maid, CapriSun, and Sunny Delight, is some form of sugar – sucrose, fructose, glucose, or sorbitol. Most have their fiber removed from them and contain high levels of sodium.

Look for products that are 100 percent fruit juice, or reconstituted juice, that are *unsweetened*. In most cases, organic juices are the best. If you can't find any, make your own juice or eat an orange or another fruit instead. There's a world of difference from your body's perspective.

If you choose to use soy, rice of another type of plant-based milk, make sure you purchase the fat free or very low-fat variety and that it does not contain oil or carrageenan (some are sensitive to this ingredient and I would recommend avoiding it).

Avoid store bought baked goods because they will likely contain hydrogenated vegetable oils, no matter how healthy they look or are advertised.

Breakfast Recipes

Barley Scones
Makes 12 scones

1 1/8 cup barley flour
1/4 cup water
3 tbsp raisins
2 tbsp maple syrup
1 tbsp applesauce (or oil substitute)
2 tsp vinegar
1 tsp baking powder
1/4 tsp baking soda

Preheat oven to 350. Mix water, maple syrup, applesauce, and vinegar. Set aside. Combine flour, baking soda and raisins in a food processor. Blend. Add liquid ingredients and process until dough forms. Transfer to flat surface, dusted with barley flour. Flatten into a circle 6 inches in diameter and 3/4 inch thick. Use knife to score dough into 12 wedges (do not separate), then transfer to a baking sheet. Bake for 30 minutes, or until lightly browned.

Black Beans with Salsa on Toast
Serves 2

1 cup dry black beans (*See Rules for Meal Preparation, Bean Preparation*)
1/4 cup diced onions
1 tsp thinly sliced jalapenos
1 large tomato, diced
4 slices of your favorite toast or tortillas
garlic powder, and cumin to taste

Heat and mash beans. For the salsa, mix the jalapenos, tomatoes, and onions, adjusting amounts to taste. Serve the beans and salsa on toast or with tortillas.

Cereal – Rolled Oats Cold

Rolled oats (not cooked)
Banana (or peach, mango, kiwis, melons, apricots, etc.)
Mixed berries
Pineapple slices
Raisins
1 tbsp ground flaxseed or flaxseed meal
Water

Pour rolled oats into bowl. Add fruits and flaxseed. Add water, to taste.

Coffee Cake
Serves 6

2 cups whole wheat flour
1 cup unsweetened apple juice
3/4 cup old-fashioned rolled oats
1/2 cup applesauce
1/2 cup maple syrup
1 tbsp baking powder
2 tsp ground cinnamon
1/2 tsp ground nutmeg
1/4 tsp ground ginger

Preheat the oven to 350. Grease 9-inch square baking pan with an oil substitute and flour. In a large bowl, add flour, 1/2 cup of oats, baking powder, cinnamon, syrup, nutmeg and ginger. Remove 1/2 cup of mixture to a cup or small bowl, add remaining 1/4 cup oats. Cut in 2 tablespoons of applesauce, set the mixture aside. Cut remaining applesauce into the flour mixture in the large bowl. Stir in the apple juice until well combined. Pour the batter into the prepared pan. Top with the reserved oat mixture. Bake about 40 minutes, or until done.

French Toast
Serves 2 to 3

2 medium bananas
2/3 water
2 tbsp maple syrup
1/8 tsp ground cinnamon
4 slices bread

Blend bananas, water, maple syrup, and cinnamon until smooth. Pour into a flat, shallow dish and soak bread slices 1 minute on each side. Transfer carefully to a skillet. Cook first side until lightly browned, about 3 minutes, then turn and cook second side until browned. Serve with fresh fruit, fruit preserves, or maple syrup.

Muffins – Apple Oat
Makes 12 medium muffins

3 cups whole wheat pastry flour
1 12-ounce can apple juice concentrate
2 large apples, finely chopped
1-1/4 cups oat bran
1/2 cup raisins
2-1/2 tsp baking soda
1 tsp ground cinnamon
1/2 tsp grated nutmeg

Preheat oven to 325. In a large bowl, mix flour, oats, spices and baking soda. Add the chopped apple along with the apple juice concentrate and raisins. Stir just enough to mix. Spoon batter into muffin tins and bake for 25 minutes.

Muffins – Pumpkin Spice
Makes 10 to 12 muffins

2 cups whole wheat pastry flour
1/2 cup maple syrup
1/2 cup raisins
1 tbsp baking powder
1/2 tsp baking soda
1/2 tsp cinnamon
1/4 tsp nutmeg
1 15-ounce can solid-pack pumpkin (or fresh)

Preheat oven to 375. Mix flour, maple syrup, baking powder, baking soda, cinnamon, and nutmeg in a large bowl. Add pumpkin, 1/2 cup water, and raisins. Stir until just mixed. Spoon batter into muffin cups. Bake 25 to 30 minutes. Remove from oven and let stand 5 minutes. Remove muffins from pan and cool.

Pancakes – Cornmeal
Makes 16 3-inch pancakes

1 cup water
1/2 cup cornmeal
1/2 cup whole wheat pastry flour
2 tbsp maple syrup
1 tbsp cider vinegar
1/2 tsp sodium-free baking powder
1/4 tsp baking soda

In a large bowl mix water, maple syrup, and vinegar. Set aside. In separate bowl stir together cornmeal, flour, baking powder, baking soda. Add to water mixture, stirring to remove any lumps and make a batter. Add more water if batter seems too thick. On skillet or griddle, pour small amounts of batter onto the heated surface and cook until tops bubble. Turn carefully with a spatula and cook the second sides until browned. Use fruit preserves, fresh fruit, or maple syrup for serving

Pancakes – Old-Fashioned
Makes 16 3-inch pancakes

1 ripe banana, mashed
1 cup water
1/2 cup buckwheat flour
1/2 cup cornmeal
2 tbsp maple syrup
1 tbsp vinegar
1/2 tsp sodium-free baking powder
1/4 tsp baking soda

Mix buckwheat flour, cornmeal, baking powder, baking soda. In a large bowl, combine mashed banana, maple syrup, vinegar, and water. Add flour mixture, stirring just enough to remove any lumps and make a batter. Add more water if batter seems too thick. On skillet or griddle, pour small amounts of batter onto the heated surface and cook until tops bubble. Turn carefully with a spatula and cook the second sides until browned. Use fruit preserves, fresh fruit, or maple syrup for serving

Granola – Maple Walnut
Makes about 6 cups

3 cups rolled oats
1 cup wheat germ
1/2 cup chopped walnuts
1/2 cup raisins
1/2 cup dried cranberries (optional)
1/4 cup sesame seeds
1/4 cup maple syrup
2 tbsp molasses
1 tsp cinnamon

Preheat oven to 300. Combine all ingredients in a large bowl and mix thoroughly. Transfer to a 9 × 13-inch baking dish. Bake, turning often with a spatula, until mixture is golden brown, about 25 minutes.

Muesli
Makes 3 cups

2 cups rolled oats
1/2 cup chopped dried fruit (apples, figs, apricots, etc.)
1/2 cup raisins

Combine all ingredients. They may be left whole or ground in a food processor until they are of a fairly fine, uniform texture. Store in an airtight container in the refrigerator. Serve with water to moisten and fresh cut fruit toppings.

Waffles – Oatmeal
Makes 6 waffles

1 banana
2 cups rolled oats
2 cups water
1 tbsp maple syrup
1 tsp vanilla

Preheat waffle iron to medium-high. Combine oats, water, banana, maple syrup and vanilla in a blender. Blend on high speed until completely smooth. Pour in batter and cook until golden brown (5-10 minutes without lifting lid.) Serve with fresh fruit.

Whole Wheat Pancakes
Makes 24 2-inch pancakes

1 banana
1 1/4 cups water
1 cup whole wheat pastry flour or whole wheat flour
1 tbsp maple syrup
2 tsp sodium-free baking powder

In a large bowl, mash banana, then stir in water and maple syrup. In a separate bowl mix flour and baking powder. Add to banana mixture and stir until smooth. Pour small amounts of batter onto a preheated griddle or skillet with a small amount of oil substitute and cook until tops bubble. Flip with a spatula and cook second side until golden brown, about 1 minute. Use fruit preserves, fresh fruit, or maple syrup for serving

Lunch or Dinner Recipes

Suggestions for Lunch/Dinner

The following are simply suggestions that you can whip up on your own without following any recipe.

Acorn squash with rice
Angel hair zucchini with marinara sauce and sweet potato or squash
Avocado, tomato, cucumber and hummus sandwich
Bean enchiladas (frozen)
Bean soup and stir-fried vegetables
Bean, vegetable and barley soup
Beets, raisins and carrots
Brown rice and vegetables
Carrot soup
Corn chowder
Corn stew
Garden salad
Garden salad wrap
Green beans and garlic mashed potatoes (keep the skins)
Lentil, tomato, etc. soup with whole wheat bread
Pasta, tomato sauce and vegetables
Pasta and vegetables
Pasta, tomato sauce and vegetables
Portobello mushroom burgers and beans
Raw vegetables
Rice and vegetables
Roasted eggplant, corn & zucchini wrap
Roasted peppers stuffed with rice and vegetables
Salad stuffed pita
Salad and raw vegetables
Soy chili
Stir-fry vegetables
Vegetable soup
Vegetable pate sandwich
Vegetarian chili

Salads

Salad - Antipasto
Makes about 6 cups

1 large red potato, scrubbed
1 carrot, sliced
1 cup Italian green beans, fresh or frozen
1 cup cauliflower florets
1 small red bell pepper, sliced or diced
2 garlic cloves, pressed
2 tbsp finely chopped parsley
2 tbsp balsamic vinegar
1 tbsp seasoned rice vinegar
1 tbsp vegetable broth
1 tbsp lemon juice
2 tsp apple juice concentrate
1 tsp stone ground or Dijon-style mustard
1/4 tsp black pepper

Dice potatoes and steam with carrots over boiling water until just tender, about 10 minutes. Place in a salad bowl. Steam green beans and cauliflower until just tender. Add to salad. Add bell pepper and parsley. Mix vinegars, vegetable broth, lemon juice, apple juice concentrate, garlic, mustard and pepper in a small bowl. Pour over vegetables, and toss to mix.

Salad – Aztec
Makes about 8 cups

3 cups dry black beans (*See Rules for Meal Preparation, Bean Preparation*)
2 tomatoes, diced
2 garlic cloves, pressed or finely minced
1 lemon or lime, juiced
1 10-ounce bag frozen corn, thawed, or 2 cups fresh corn
3/4 cup chopped fresh cilantro (optional)
1/2 cup finely chopped red onion
1 green bell pepper, seeded and diced
1 red or yellow bell pepper, seeded and diced
2 tbsp seasoned rice vinegar
2 tbsp apple cider or distilled vinegar
2 tsp ground cumin
1 tsp coriander

1/2 tsp red pepper flakes or a pinch of cayenne

In a large bowl, combine beans, onion, bell peppers, corn, tomatoes, and cilantro. In a small bowl, whisk together vinegars, lemon juice, garlic, cumin, coriander, and red pepper flakes. Pour over salad and toss gently to mix.

Salad – Black Bean & Corn

3 cups dry black beans (*See Rules for Meal Preparation, Bean Preparation*)
2 cups frozen corn kernels, thawed
2 tomatoes, chopped
1 red pepper, chopped
1 jalapeno pepper, minced
1 cup chopped green onions
1/2 cup chopped red onion
1/2 cup chopped cilantro
1-2 tbsp Juice from 1 lime
1 tbsp vegetable broth
1 tsp minced garlic

Combine first seven ingredients in a large bowl. Make dressing with lime juice, cilantro, garlic, pepper and vegetable broth. Combine well. Pour over salad ingredients and toss lightly to combine. Chill several hours before serving.

Salad – Black-eyed Peas Salad
Makes about 5 cups

2 cups cooked black-eyed peas
1-1/2 cups cooked brown rice
1 celery stalk, thinly sliced (about 1/2 cup)
1 tomato, diced
1/2 cup finely sliced green onions
2 tbsp finely chopped parsley

Combine the above ingredients in a mixing bowl. Add no-oil salad dressing.

Salad – Broccoli
Makes about 4 cups

1 bunch broccoli
1–2 garlic cloves, minced
1/2 cup finely sliced red onion
1/2 cup seasoned rice vinegar
1 tbsp vegetable broth
1/2 tsp dried red pepper flakes

Cut or break broccoli into small florets. Transfer to a salad bowl. Add remaining ingredients and toss to mix. Chill, tossing once or twice, for 20 minutes or longer before serving.

Salad – Colorful
Serves 4

1 sweet red pepper, cut into chunks
1 orange
1 cup of snap peas, cut in half
1 cucumber, peeled and cut into chunks
8 fresh basil leaves, sliced
1 tbsp seasoned rice vinegar
cracked black pepper, to taste

Remove the peel off the orange and cut the peeled fruit into bite size chunks. In medium bowl, mix together the orange, red pepper, cucumber, and basil. Sprinkle with rice vinegar and season with pepper. Toss and serve.

Salad – Crunchy
Serves 6

1 15-ounce can diced beets, drained
2 medium-size carrots, peeled and cut into thin strips or diced
1 small jicama, peeled and cut into thin strips or diced
3 tbsp of lemon juice
2 tbsp seasoned rice vinegar
2 tsp stone ground mustard
1/2 tsp dried dill weed

Place beet cubes into a large salad bowl, along with jicama and carrot pieces. In a small bowl, mix lemon juice, vinegar, mustard, and dill; pour over the salad. Toss to mix. Serve warm or chilled.

Salad – Cucumber Arame
Serves 4 to 6

1 cucumber
1 cup arame
1 cup water
2 tbsp lemon juice
2 tbsp water
1 tbsp brown rice vinegar
1 tsp low-sodium Tamari (soy sauce)

Peel and halve the cucumber lengthwise. Transfer to a bowl and let stand 15 minutes. Drain thoroughly. Meanwhile, soak the arame in one cup of water until soft, 10 to 15 minutes. Mix together lemon juice, Tamari, vinegar and 2 tablespoons of water to make dressing. Drain any excess water from arame, then combine with cucumber and dressing.

Salad – Cucumber, Mango & Spinach
Serves 10-12

1 bag or bunch of spinach
1 mango, peeled and cut into bite size pieces
1 large English cucumber, peeled and sliced
6 scallions, thinly sliced
1/2 cup fresh, chopped basil leaves
Juice of 1 lime
1/2 cup seasoned rice vinegar
Fresh cracked black pepper to taste

Wash and drain spinach, tear into bite-sized pieces if necessary, and put into a large serving bowl. Toss mango, cucumber, scallions, and basil in a medium bowl. Dress with lime juice and vinegar. Arrange mango mixture on spinach and sprinkle with fresh cracked black pepper.

Salad – Fiesta
Serves 10

4 cups dry black beans (*See Rules for Meal Preparation, Bean Preparation*)
2 cups frozen corn, thawed
2 large tomatoes, diced
1 large green bell pepper, diced
1 large red or yellow bell pepper, diced
3/4 cups chopped cilantro
1/2 cup chopped red onion

Combine beans with the corn, tomatoes, bell peppers, red onion, and cilantro. Toss with no-oil dressing.

Salad – Mediterranean Rice Salad
Serves 6 to 8

3 Roma tomatoes, cut into chunks
3 cups cooked brown rice
1 green pepper, chopped
1 cucumber, peeled and cut into chunks
1 cup green beans, broken into small pieces, blanched or raw
1/2 cup fresh basil leaves, sliced
1/2 cup seasoned rice vinegar
1 tbsp mustard
1 tbsp vegetable broth
1/2 tsp dried parsley flakes
juice of 1 lemon

In medium bowl, mix together rice, pepper, green beans, cucumber, tomato, and basil. Stir together mustard, rice vinegar, lemon juice, vegetable broth, and parsley. Pour over salad and toss to mix. Season with pepper. Toss and serve.

Salad – Mixed Greens with Apples & Walnuts
Makes about 4 cups

6 cups salad mix or washed and torn butter lettuce
1 tart green apple (Granny Smith, pippin, or similar)
1/4 cup chopped walnuts
3-4 tbsp seasoned rice vinegar

Place salad mix or torn leaf lettuce into a bowl. Core and dice apple and add to salad along with walnuts. Sprinkle with seasoned rice vinegar and toss to mix.

Salad – Pasta Salad
Serves 8-10

12 ounces pasta shells (about 2 cups)
1 jar water-packed artichoke hearts, drained and quartered
2-3 cups button mushrooms (about 1/2 pound)
1 garlic clove
1 small red bell pepper, diced
1/2 cup chopped green onions
1/3 cup seasoned rice vinegar
1/4 cup cider vinegar
3 tbsp water
3 tbsp chopped fresh parsley
2 tbsp fresh lemon juice (optional)
2 tsp stone-ground or Dijon-style mustard
1/2 tsp each dried basil and oregano
1/4 tsp black pepper

Cook until pasta is tender. Rinse, drain, place in a large bowl. Add artichoke hearts and mushrooms. In a blender, combine the vinegars, lemon juice, mustard, 1/4 cup green onions, garlic, seasonings, and water. Process until smooth. Pour over pasta, and allow to marinate until pasta is cool. Add the remaining green onions, parsley, and red bell pepper and gently toss to mix.

Salad – Rice Salad

3 cups cooked brown rice
3 Roma tomatoes, cut into chunks
1 green, yellow or red pepper, chopped
1 cucumber, peeled and cut into chunks
1 cup raw green beans, cut into small pieces
1/2 cup basil leaves, sliced
1/2 cup seasoned rice vinegar
1 tbsp mustard
1/2 tsp dried parsley flakes
1/2 tsp Italian seasoning
juice of 1 lemon

In bowl, mix together rice, pepper, green beans, cucumber, tomato, and basil. Stir together mustard, rice vinegar, lemon juice and parsley. Pour over salad and toss to mix. Season with pepper and Tabasco (optional) to taste. Toss and serve.

Salad – Spanish Wild Rice

2 cups wild rice
Dried apricots, diced
Walnuts, chopped
Juice from one orange
Spring onions, chopped
Balsamic vinegar

Cook rice with water and orange juice until done, but still a little firm. Toss in some dried apricots, walnuts and spring onions. Pour Balsamic vinegar to taste over the rice and chill.

Salad – Spinach
Serves 2

2 cups spinach
1/2 cup sliced mushrooms
1/4 cup chopped green onions
Tamari (optional)
Sesame seeds, for garnish

Thoroughly wash the spinach, tearing the larger leaves. Drain well. Add the mushrooms and green onions, and toss well. Sprinkle with Tamari, if desired, then sprinkle each serving with sesame seeds.

Salad – Spinach with Fruit
Serves 4

4 cups cleaned spinach leaves
2 oranges, peeled, sliced, and quartered
1 cucumber, peeled, sliced and quartered
1 sweet red pepper, seeded and chopped
2 tbsp raw or roasted sunflower seeds

Toss spinach with cucumber, orange, and red pepper chunks in medium sized bowl. Sprinkle with sunflower seeds. Serve with no-oil dressing on the side.

Salad – Squash, Corn & Bean Salad
Makes about 8 cups

15 ounces fresh or frozen corn
2 cups black beans (*See Rules for Meal Preparation, Bean Preparation*)
1 red bell pepper, diced
2 cups butternut or kabocha squash, julienne or cut into 1/4-inch cubes (available frozen in health food stores)
1 cup jicama, julienne or cut into 1/4-inch cubes
1/2 cup red onion
1/2 cup chopped cilantro
1/4 cup pumpkin seeds
1/4 cup seasoned rice vinegar
2 tbsp lemon or lime juice
1 tsp each: cumin, coriander, chili powder
1 garlic clove, pressed or minced

Combine squash, jicama, bell pepper, corn, beans, onion, cilantro and pumpkin seeds in a large bowl.
Mix vinegar, lemon juice, cumin, coriander, chili powder and garlic. Pour over salad and toss to mix.

Salad – Stuffed Tomato
Serves 5

5 large ripe tomatoes
2 cups dry garbanzo beans (*See Rules for Meal Preparation, Bean Preparation*)
1 stalk celery, chopped (optional)

Scoop out tomatoes, saving pulp for a sauce. Fill tomatoes with beans and celery. Season with pepper. Garnish with sauce and lettuce or sprouts.

Salad – Three Bean
Serves 4

(See Rules for Meal Preparation, Bean Preparation)
2 cups dry kidney beans
2 cups dry garbanzo beans
2 cups dry lima beans
1 cup onion, chopped
1/2 cup green pepper, chopped
4 tsp vegetable broth

Toss ingredients together. Serve hot or cold with a grain or bread. To serve cold for a salad, add a few drops of lemon juice or vinegar.

Salad – Tomato, Cucumber & Basil
Serves 6

4 fresh tomatoes, quartered and sliced
1/2 large English cucumber, peeled, quartered and sliced
1/2 cup fresh basil leaves,
3-4 tbsp balsamic vinegar

Arrange cucumber and tomato in a flat bowl. Add basil leaves, dress with balsamic vinegar, and sprinkle with fresh cracked black pepper.

Salad – White Bean
Makes about 2 1/2 cups

2 cups dry white beans *(See Rules for Meal Preparation, Bean Preparation)*
1 small red bell pepper, diced
1/2 cup finely chopped fresh parsley
1 lemon, juiced
2 tsp balsamic vinegar
1/4 tsp garlic granules or powder
1/4 tsp black pepper

Combine all ingredients in a large bowl and toss to mix. Let stand 10 to 15 minutes before serving.

Soups & Stews

Chowder – Kale and Rice
Serves 6

2 cups, diced stewed tomatoes
2 cups vegetable broth
2 cups chopped kale
1 cup cooked brown rice
2 cups dry garbanzo beans (*See Rules for Meal Preparation, Bean Preparation*)
1 cup chopped onion
1 cup chopped red bell pepper
1 1/2 cups water
1/2 cup chopped leeks
1/3 cup sliced almonds
1 tbsp paprika
2 tsp vegetable broth for sautéing
2 bay leaves

Heat the broth over medium-high heat. Add the onion, pepper, leeks, and almonds. Sauté for 2 minutes. Add the almonds, paprika, bay leaves, water, tomatoes, and broth. Bring to boil. Add the kale, rice, and garbanzo beans. Reduce heat and simmer 10 minutes, or until thoroughly heated.

Soup – Black Bean Creamy
Serves 4 to 6

3 cloves garlic, crushed
6-7 cups water
2-1/2 cups (1 pound) dried black beans
1 cup water
1 tbsp vegetable broth
tortillas for garnish (whole wheat)
lettuce for garnish

Soak beans overnight. Drain and cover with water. Add the garlic and cook until soft, about 2 hours, or five minutes in a pressure cooker. Blend beans with the cooking water and return to pot. Reheat with vegetable broth and water. Garnish with thinly sliced fried tortillas and strips of lettuce.

Soup – Carrot and Red Pepper
Serves 4

6 carrots, thinly sliced
2 red bell peppers, roasted
1 onion, chopped
2 cups water
2 cups water or vegetable stock
2 tsp lemon juice
2 tsp balsamic vinegar
1/4 tsp freshly ground black pepper

Place the chopped onion and carrots into a pot with the water and simmer, covered, over medium heat until the carrots can be easily pierced with a fork, about 20 minutes. Roast the peppers by placing them over an open gas flame or directly under the broiler. Place in a bowl, cover, and let stand about 15 minutes. Cut the peppers in half and remove the seeds. Blend the carrot mixture along with the peppers in several small batches. Add some of the water to each batch to facilitate blending. Return to the pot and add the lemon juice, vinegar and pepper. Heat until steamy.

Soup – Chilled Cucumber-Dill
Makes 1 serving

1-1/2 cups water
1/2 cucumber
1 tbsp fresh dill weed or 1 tsp dried dill weed

Chill the water in the freezer for 15 minutes. Put the cucumber through a juicer. Combine the cucumber juice and water in a blender. Pour into a bowl and top with the dill weed.

Soup – Cream of Asparagus
Makes about 7 cups

2 medium-size white potatoes, diced
1 medium-size bunch asparagus (about 4 cups chopped)
2 cups water
2 cups shredded cabbage
1-2 cups water
1 cup (loosely packed) chopped fresh parsley
1/4 cup chopped fresh basil

Dice potatoes (do not peel them). Place them into a large pot with the water. Bring to a simmer, cover and cook until tender. Remove the tough ends from the asparagus, then break stalks into 1- to 2-inch lengths. When potatoes are tender, add asparagus along with cabbage, parsley, and basil. Cover and simmer for about 5 minutes, or until asparagus is just tender when pierced with a fork. In a blender purée the vegetables with cooking liquid, in 2 or 3 batches. Add enough of the water to each batch to facilitate blending. After puréeing all vegetables, pour soup into the pan, then heat gently until steamy.

Soup – Creamy Beet
Makes about 3 cups

1 15-ounce can diced beets
1 cup water
2 tbsp apple juice concentrate
1 tsp balsamic vinegar
1/2 tsp dried dill weed

Place diced beets, water, apple juice concentrate, vinegar, and dill weed into blender. Blend on high speed until completely smooth. Transfer to a medium saucepan and heat gently until steamy. Serve hot or cold.

Soup – Curried Potato and Onion
Serves 6

2 medium onions, chopped
2 large garlic cloves, pressed or minced
4-1/2 cups vegetable broth or bouillon
2 to 3 cups peeled and diced potatoes
3/4 cup water
2 tsp vegetable broth
1-1/2 tsp ground cumin
1-1/2 tsp curry powder, or to taste
1 tsp ground tumeric
chopped fresh chives or cilantro for garnish

In a large soup pot, sauté the garlic and onion in the broth until transparent. Add spices and 1/4 cup broth; stir well and cook for 5 minutes. Add the potatoes and remaining broth. Simmer gently for 20 minutes, or until potatoes are soft. Purée in batches in a food processor or use a hand held blender and blend until smooth. If serving cold, refrigerate for at least 6 hours.

Soup – Curried Sweet Potato
Serves 6

5 cups cubed, peeled sweet potato
4 cups vegetable broth
1 cup chopped onion
1 cup water
1/8 cup vegetable broth
2 tsp curry powder
minced cilantro (optional)

Heat broth in a large saucepan over medium heat. Add the onion and curry powder and sauté for 2 minutes. Add the water, broth, and sweet potatoes. Cook for 30 minutes, or until the sweet potatoes are tender. Place one-third of the sweet potato mixture in a blender and process until smooth. Repeat the procedure with the remaining sweet potato mixture in batches. Return the puréed mixture to the saucepan. Bring the soup to a boil and remove from heat. Garnish with cilantro, if desired.

Soup – Gazpacho
Serves 4

1 plum tomato, seeded and finely diced
2 garlic cloves, chopped
2 cups tomato juice
1/4 cup seeded and diced cucumber
1/4 cup finely diced green bell pepper
1/4 cup red onion, finely diced
1/4 cup zucchini, finely diced (optional)
4 tbs. vegetable broth
2 tbs. bread crumbs
1 tbs. white wine vinegar

Place the tomato juice, garlic and broth in a blender and process until the garlic is puréed. Add the bread crumbs and vinegar, and blend to combine. Add favorite seasonings. Pour into a covered container and chill well, from 2 hours to overnight. When ready to serve, check the seasoning and adjust if necessary. Divide the soup among 4 serving bowls. Add 1 Tbs. each of the diced cucumber, pepper, tomato and onion, plus the zucchini if desired.

Soup – Lentil
Serves 8

2 onions, halved and sliced
4 cloves garlic, minced
3 parsnips, peeled and sliced
10 cups water
5 cups packed chopped dandelion greens or kale
2 cups red lentils, rinsed and drained
1/8 cup vegetable broth
1 5 ounce can tomato paste
3 tbsp chopped parsley, divided
1 tsp dried oregano
1 tsp dried basil
1 tsp black pepper

In a large pot, heat vegetable broth over medium-high heat. Add onions and sauté for 3 minutes. Add garlic and sauté 1 minute more. Add water, lentils, tomato paste, parsnips, 1 tablespoon parsley, oregano, basil, and pepper. Bring to a boil. Reduce heat to low, cover and simmer for 30 minutes. Add dandelion greens and simmer an additional 15 minutes or until greens are soft. Garnish with remaining parsley.

Soup – Minestrone
Makes about 2 1/2 quarts

2 cups dry kidney beans (*See Rules for Meal Preparation, Bean Preparation*)
1 small onion, chopped
1 carrot, cut into chunks
1 celery stalk, sliced including top
1 potato, scrubbed and cut into chunks
1 small zucchini, diced
4 garlic cloves, minced
2 cups tomato juice
2 cups water or vegetable broth
1 cup finely chopped kale, collard greens, or spinach
2 tbsp chopped parsley
1/4 tsp black pepper
1/4 cup pasta shells
1 tbsp chopped fresh basil or 1 tsp dried basil
1 tsp mixed Italian herbs

Combine onion, garlic, carrot, celery, potato, and parsley in a large pot. Add tomato juice, water or broth, Italian herbs, and black pepper. Bring to a simmer, then cover and cook 20 minutes. Add zucchini, pasta, kidney beans, chopped greens, and basil. Cover and simmer until pasta is tender, about 20 minutes. Add extra tomato juice or water for a thinner soup.

Soup – Mushroom and Barley
Makes about 3 cups

2 cups water
1 cup cooked barley
1 4-ounce can mushrooms, including the liquid
2 tbsp barley flour
1/4 tsp garlic powder
pinch each of dried marjoram, sage, thyme, and dill weed

Place water and barley flour into blender. Blend on high speed for a few seconds. Add barley and blend until barley is chopped coarse. Add mushrooms with their liquid. Blend just enough to coarse-chop mushrooms. Transfer the blended mixture to a medium-sized saucepan and add all the remaining ingredients. Cook over medium heat until soup is hot and somewhat thickened.

Soup – Split Pea & Barley
Makes 8-9 cups

2 quarts water
1 carrot, chopped
3 stalks celery, diced
1 potato, diced
1 onion, diced
1 cup green split peas
1/4 cup barley
1 tsp celery seed
1/2 tsp basil
1/2 tsp thyme

Sauté onion until soft in a little water, along with the celery seed. Stir in peas and barley. Add water and bring to a boil. Cook on low heat, partially covered, for about an hour and a half. Add pepper, vegetable and herbs. Simmer another 30 to 45 minutes.

Soup – Vegetable Soup with Hominy
Serves 4

1 15-ounce can of white hominy
1 1/2 cups stewed tomatoes with garlic, green pepper, and celery
4 carrots, sliced
3 cloves garlic, minced
1 large onion, chopped
1 red pepper, chopped
3 cups of water or low-sodium vegetable stock
1 cup green beans, broken into bite-sized lengths
3/4 tsp chili powder
1/2 tsp cumin
1/4 tsp pepper

In medium stock pot, braise garlic and onion in 1/2 cup water until soft. Add carrots and water or stock, and simmer 5 to 10 minutes. Drain and rinse hominy and add to the pot. Stir in the tomatoes, red pepper, green beans, and spices. Simmer for 15 minutes. Serve piping hot with little bowls of the toppings. Use salsa or chopped lettuce as toppings.

Stew – Green Split Pea and Barley

3 garlic cloves
2 large white potatoes, coarsely chopped
2 stalks celery, diced
2 large carrots, diced
6 cups water
2 cups chopped fresh spinach
1 medium yellow onion -- diced
1 cup green split peas -- rinsed
1/2 cup pearl barley
2 tbsp dried parsley
2 tbsp vegetable broth
2 tsp dried oregano or thyme leaves
1/2 tsp black pepper

In a large saucepan, heat the broth over medium heat. Add the onion, celery, carrots, and garlic and cook, stirring, for about 7 minutes. Add the water, split peas, barley, potatoes, parsley, oregano, and pepper and bring to a simmer over medium-high heat. Reduce the heat to medium and cook until peas are tender, about 1 hour. Stir in the spinach and cook over low heat for 10 to 15 minutes. Ladle into bowls and serve with warm whole wheat bread. (Note: To speed up the cooking time, soak the split peas in water for 1 hour before cooking.)

Stew – Lentil and Barley Stew
Makes about 1 1/2 quarts

1 small onion, chopped
1 garlic clove, pressed or minced
1 carrot, diced
1 celery stalk, sliced
1 quart vegetable broth or water
1/2 cup lentils, rinsed
1/4 cup hulled or pearled barley
1/2 tsp oregano
1/2 tsp ground cumin
1/4 tsp red pepper flakes
1/4 tsp black pepper

Place all ingredients into a large pot and bring to a simmer. Cover and cook, stirring occasionally, until lentils and barley are tender, about 1 hour.

Stew – Spicy Pumpkin
Serves 6

2 cups dry red kidney or pinto beans (*See Rules for Meal Preparation, Bean Preparation*)
1 cup fresh or frozen corn kernels
1 medium onion, thinly sliced
3-4 cups of small chunk (1/2-inch) raw pumpkin or butternut squash
1 cup vegetable stock
1 cup tomato sauce
1/2 cup salsa
1 tsp minced garlic
1 tsp chili powder
1/2 tsp hot red pepper flakes
1/2 tsp cumin
3-4 drops of Tabasco

Simmer pumpkin or squash in vegetable stock until tender. Add remaining ingredients and simmer uncovered over low heat for 30 minutes. Season to taste.

Stew – Summer
Makes about 2 1/2 quarts

2 cups dry cannelini beans or navy beans (*See Rules for Meal Preparation, Bean Preparation*)
1 12-ounce jar water-packed roasted red peppers, including liquid
5 large garlic cloves, minced
2 onions, chopped
4 cups eggplant, cut into 1/4-inch thick slices
3 cups zucchini, sliced
2 cups chopped fresh basil
1 green bell pepper, diced
1 cup water or vegetable broth
2 tbsp vegetable broth
1/4 tsp black pepper

Heat broth in a large pot, add onions. Cook over medium heat until onions are lightly browned. Add a small amounts of water if onions begin to stick. Add eggplant, bell pepper, and garlic, then cover and cook five minutes.. Coarsely chop red peppers and add, with their liquid. Add zucchini, basil, and water. Cover and cook over medium heat, stirring occasionally, for 3 minutes. Stir in cannelini beans, including liquid, and black pepper. Cover and cook until zucchini is just tender, about 3 minutes.

Mix-Ins/Side Dishes

Asparagus with Garlic & Pecans
Serves 4

1 pound asparagus, broken into bite-sized pieces
3 cloves garlic, minced
1/2 cup pecans, halved
1 tbsp low-sodium Tamari (soy sauce)
2 tsp vegetable broth

Sauté garlic in broth in medium skillet. Add asparagus and Tamari. Cook 4-6 minutes stirring often until asparagus is tender. Add pecans, continue heating for 1-2 minutes and serve.

Asparagus with Raspberry Sauce
Serves 4

1 pound of asparagus
1 cup frozen raspberries
1/2 fresh orange or 1 tsp frozen orange juice concentrate
1 tsp orange zest (optional)

Put frozen raspberries in saucepot with orange juice or juice concentrate. Simmer until raspberries have fallen apart and mixture looks like a sauce. Remove from heat and set aside. Steam asparagus over hot water until just tender.. Pour sauce over asparagus. Serve hot or at room temperature. Garnish with orange zest, if desired.

Beans – Baked Beans
Makes about 8 cups

(*See Rules for Meal Preparation, Bean Preparation*)
2-1/2 cups dry navy beans (or other small white beans)
1 onion, chopped
2-1/2 cups dried navy beans (or other small white beans)
1/2 cup molasses
2 tbsp vinegar
2 tsp stone ground or Dijon mustard
1 tsp Bakkon yeast (optional – found at health food stores)
1/2 tsp garlic granules or powder

Place beans in a large pot with onion. Add tomato sauce, molasses, mustard, vinegar, garlic granules and Bakkon yeast if using. Cook, loosely covered, over very low heat for 1 to 2 hours. Or, transfer to an ovenproof dish and bake at 350 for 2 to 3 hours.

Beans – Barbecued
Makes 6 cups

(*See Rules for Meal Preparation, Bean Preparation*)
2 cups dry pinto beans
2 cups dry kidney beans
1 10-ounce package frozen baby lima beans
1/2 cup crushed tomatoes
1 cup finely chopped onion
1 tbsp cider vinegar
1 tbsp molasses
2 tsp stone-ground mustard
1 tsp chili powder

Combine all ingredients in a saucepan and cook at a slow simmer for 25 to 30 minutes.

Beans – Black Beans and Tomatoes
Makes 4 cups

4 cups dry black beans (*See Rules for Meal Preparation, Bean Preparation*)
4 cups diced tomatoes
2 garlic cloves, minced
1/2 cup chopped onion
1/4 cup vegetable broth
2 tbsp canned, chopped green chilies
1 tbsp chopped cilantro or parsley
1/2 tsp cumin
1/2 tsp ground red pepper
1/4 tsp chili powder

Heat 1/4-cup vegetable broth in cooking skillet and heat over medium-high heat. Add chopped onion and garlic. Sauté in broth until tender. Add tomatoes and chilies. Reduce heat and cook uncovered 6 to 8 minutes or until mixture is slightly thickened, stirring occasionally. Stir in beans and remaining ingredients. Cover and cook five minutes or until thoroughly heated.

Beans – Refried Beans (spicy)
Makes about 5 cups

1 1/2 cups dry pinto beans
1 onion, chopped
1 cup crushed or finely chopped tomatoes
1 4-ounce can diced green chilies
4 garlic cloves, minced or pressed
1 1/2 tsp cumin
1/4 tsp cayenne

Clean and rinse beans, then soak in about 6 cups of water for 6 to 8 hours. Discard soaking water, rinse beans and place in a large pot with 4 cups fresh water, minced garlic, cumin, and cayenne. Simmer until tender, about 1 hour. Heat 1/2 cup of water in a large skillet. Add onion and cook until soft, about 5 minutes. Stir in tomatoes and diced chilies. Cook, uncovered, over medium heat for 10 minutes, stirring occasionally. Add cooked beans, including some cooking liquid, a cup at a time to tomato mixture. Mash some of the beans as you add them. When all the beans have been added, stir to mix, then cook over low heat, stirring frequently, until thickened.

Beets in Dill Sauce
Makes about 4 cups

4 medium-sized beets
2 tbsp lemon juice
1 tbsp stone-ground mustard
1 tbsp cider vinegar
1 tbsp apple juice concentrate
1 tsp dried dill weed, or 1 tbsp fresh dill, chopped

Wash and peel the beets, then slice them into 1/4-inch thick rounds. Steam over boiling water until tender when pierced with a fork, about 20 minutes. Mix the remaining ingredients in a serving bowl. Add the beets and toss to mix. Serve immediately, or chill before serving.

Barley Cakes – Spinach
Makes 10 barley cakes

1 10-ounce package frozen spinach
1 small onion
2 medium garlic cloves
1 small carrot
2 cups fresh mushrooms
2 cups cooked barley
4 tbsp vegetable broth
2 tbsp shelled sunflower seeds

Grind the sunflower seeds in a food processor. Add the onion, garlic, carrot, and mushrooms. Grind thoroughly and then add the remaining ingredients and process for about 1 minute, or until well mixed. Preheat a large, skillet. Form the barley mixture into patties. Cook each side over medium-high heat for about 3 minutes, or until golden brown.

Broccoli and Ginger (sautéed)
Serves 4

1 clove garlic, minced
1 medium leek, sliced thin (white part only)
1/2-inch piece fresh ginger root, peeled and grated
1 pound broccoli, cut into florets
2 tbsp vegetable stock
4 tsp vegetable broth
1 tsp low-sodium Tamari

Sauté the garlic and ginger in the broth in a large skillet for 1 minute. Add the broccoli, leek, and stock. Toss together all the ingredients to mix well. Cover the pan and cook for 3 minutes. Remove the cover and continue to sauté, stirring frequently, until the vegetables are just tender, about 10 minutes.

Bruschetta
Makes 1-1/2 cups

1 cup diced tomatoes, hearts discarded
2 garlic cloves, minced
1/4 cup diced red onion
1/4 cup minced fresh parsley
1/4 cup fresh basil, minced

Combine ingredients in glass or ceramic pan. Refrigerate until ready to serve. To serve, spoon onto thin slices of toasted whole wheat bread.

Buckwheat and Cabbage
Makes about 2½ cups

2 cups finely chopped cabbage
1 cup vegetable broth or water
1/2 cup buckwheat groats
4 tsp vegetable broth for sautéing

Heat broth in a large saucepan. Add kasha and shredded cabbage and cook over medium-high heat, stirring constantly, for 1 minute. Stir in 1 cup vegetable broth. Cover and simmer until buckwheat is tender and all the liquid is absorbed, about 10 minutes.

Collards or Kale – Braised
Makes 3 cups

1 bunch collard greens or kale (6 to 8 cups chopped)
2-3 garlic cloves, minced
1/4 cup water
2 tsp vegetable broth
2 tsp low-sodium Tamari (soy sauce)
1 tsp balsamic vinegar

Wash greens, remove stems, then chop leaves into 1/2-inch wide strips. Combine broth, Tamari, vinegar, garlic, and water in a large pot or skillet. Cook over high heat about 30 seconds. Reduce heat to medium-high, add chopped greens, and toss to mix. Cover and cook, stirring often, until greens are tender, about 5 minutes.

Cornbread
Serves 8

1-1/2 cups water
1 cup cornmeal
1 cup whole wheat pastry flour
4 tbsp vegetable broth
1-1/2 tbsp vinegar
2 tbsp maple syrup
1 tsp baking powder
1/2 tsp baking soda

Preheat oven to 425. Combine water and vinegar and let stand. Mix dry ingredients and maple syrup in a large bowl. Add the water mixture and the broth and stir until blended. Spread the batter into a 9-inch square baking dish and bake for 25 to 30 minutes or until done. Serve hot.

Crostini (herbed bread) with Roasted Red Peppers
Makes 1 baguette (about 20 slices)

10 sun-dried tomato halves
1 garlic clove, pressed
1 small whole wheat baguette, cut into 1/2-inch thick slices
1 cup boiling water
2/3 cup roasted red peppers (about 2 peppers)
2 tbsp fresh basil, finely chopped OR
1 tsp dried basil
1/8 tsp black pepper

Pour boiling water over tomatoes and set aside until softened, about 10 minutes. Drain and chop coarsely. Chop roasted red peppers and add to tomatoes, along with garlic, basil, and black pepper. Let stand 30 minutes. Preheat oven to 350. Slice baguette and arrange slices in a single layer on one or two baking sheets. Toast in preheated oven until outsides are crisp, 10 to 15 minutes. Remove from oven and cool slightly, then spread each piece with 1 to 2 tablespoons of tomato mixture.

Curried – Cauliflower with Peas (spicy)
Makes about 6 cups

1 10-ounce bag frozen peas
1 large onion, chopped
1 cauliflower, cut or broken into florets (about 4 cups)
1/2 cup vegetable broth or water
1-2 tbsp low-sodium Tamari (soy sauce)
1 tsp coriander
1 tsp whole mustard seed
1/2 tsp each: turmeric, cumin
1/4 tsp each: cinnamon, ginger, cardamom, cayenne pepper

Combine coriander, mustard seed, turmeric, cumin, cinnamon, ginger, cardamom, and cayenne in a large skillet. Heat, stirring constantly, until spices darken slightly and just begin to smoke: about one minute. Remove from heat and cool slightly. Add vegetable broth, Tamari, and onion. Cook until onion is soft, stirring occasionally, about five minutes. Stir in cauliflower, then cover and cook over medium heat until tender when pierced with a fork, about five minutes. Stir in peas and cook until hot, another minute or two. For a less spicy taste, cut back on the cayenne pepper. Carrots and potatoes are optional.

Curried – Chickpea
Makes 8 to 10 servings

2 cups tomato sauce
4 cans of chickpeas, drained
8 cloves garlic, minced
2 1/2 medium onions, thinly sliced
2 green peppers, cut into small pieces
1/8 cup vegetable broth
2 tsp turmeric
1 tsp cumin
1 tsp allspice
1 1/2 tsp cayenne pepper
1/2 tsp ginger

Sauté the onions in the broth. When brown, add the tomato sauce, garlic and the spices and sauté for a few minutes. Add the chickpeas and the green peppers and sauté over fairly high heat until everything is browned, about 15 minutes. Add water, if needed, turn down the heat and cover. Simmer for about 1 hour, stirring frequently. Serve over rice.

Curried – Vegetables

1 1/2 cups tomatoes, diced
4 cardamoms, bruised
2 medium zucchinis, cut into 1 inch chunks
2 bay leaves
1 small onion, peeled and finely chopped
1 large potato, peeled and diced
1 small cauliflower, stalks removed and florets divided up
1/2 cup green beans
1/4 pint hot water
1 tbsp vegetable broth
1 tbsp turmeric
1 tsp fenugreek seeds
1 tsp coriander seeds
1/2 tsp mustard seeds
1/4 tsp freshly milled black pepper

Put onion into a very large bowl with broth and sautee until onions start to brown. Add the cardamoms, fenugreek, mustard, coriander seeds and turmeric and stir occasionally. Add the diced potato to the mixture until almost cooked. Add the zucchinis, cauliflower florets, beans, tomatoes and bay leaves and add about half the water. Reduce heat and cook until the vegetables are tender, adding the remaining water if necessary. Adjust seasoning to taste.

Garlic Bread
Makes about 20 slices

2 roasted garlic heads
1 loaf whole wheat French (or other) bread, sliced
1–2 tsp mixed Italian herbs

Preheat oven to 350. Peel roasted cloves or squeeze flesh from skin and place in a bowl. Mash with a fork, then mix in Italian herbs. Spread on sliced bread. Wrap tightly in foil and bake for 20 minutes.

Green Beans – Italian Style
Makes about 6 cups

1 pound fresh green beans
2 cups chopped tomatoes, fresh or canned
2 large garlic cloves, minced
1 tbsp vegetable broth
2 tbsp chopped fresh basil or 1 tsp dried basil

Trim ends off beans and cut or break into bite-sized lengths. Steam until just tender, about 10 minutes, then set aside. Heat vegetable broth in a large skillet, then add tomatoes and garlic. Simmer 10 minutes. Add green beans and basil. Cook until beans are very tender, about 5 minutes, stirring occasionally. Season to taste.

Green Beans with Basil
Serves 4

1 lb. fresh or frozen green beans
1 tbsp minced onion
1 tsp vegetable broth
1 tsp dried basil leaves
1 tsp garlic powder
Dash pepper

Trim and snap green beans into thirds. Mince the onion. Put water on to boil to steam beans for 12-17 minutes or until tender. Sauté the onions in vegetable broth until tender. Add steamed beans, basil, garlic powder and pepper. Toss beans with basil sauce to coat evenly and serve.

Lentil–Bulgur Pilaf
6 servings

1 medium onion, minced
2 1/2 cups water
1 cup lentils
1 cup uncooked bulgur
1/2 cup minced fresh parsley
3 tbsp vegetable broth
1/2 tsp ground cumin
1/8 tsp cayenne pepper

Place lentils in a large saucepan. Add water and bring to a boil. Reduce heat, cover, and simmer for 15 minutes. Remove from heat. Stir in bulgur, cover, and set aside for 20 minutes, until bulgur is tender. Drain excess liquid. Heat broth in a skillet over medium heat. Add onion and sauté until lightly golden. Combine lentil-bulgur mixture, onion, parsley, cayenne pepper, and cumin in a large bowl and mix well.

Lentils – French Green
Makes about 6 cups

1 large onion, chopped
4 cups vegetable broth
1 cup French green lentils
1/2 cup chopped cilantro
1 tsp black mustard seeds
1 tsp turmeric
1 tsp cumin
1 tsp coriander
1/2 tsp ginger
1/4 tsp cayenne

Rinse lentils and place in a large pot with vegetable broth, onion and cilantro. Combine mustard seeds, turmeric, cumin, coriander, ginger, and cayenne in a small skillet. Toast over medium-high heat, stirring constantly, until spices are fragrant and just begin to smoke, about 2 minutes. Add to lentils. Cover and simmer until lentils are tender, about 30 minutes.

Mushrooms – In Barbeque Sauce
Serves 4

1 12-ounce package button or cremini mushrooms, sliced
1 small yellow onion, finely chopped
1/2 cup barbeque sauce

Braise onions in 1/4-cup water for 3-4 minutes. Add mushrooms and continue cooking for 4-5 more minutes. Add barbeque sauce and cook until sauce is desired thickness. Serve over veggie burgers, potatoes, or rice.

Polenta (cornmeal)
Makes 4 cups

4 cups water
1 cup polenta or stone-ground yellow cornmeal
1/2 tsp crushed dried rosemary (optional)

Bring water to a boil, then slowly pour in the polenta, stirring constantly with a whisk to prevent it from lumping. Lower heat and simmer, stirring fairly constantly until thick, about 10 minutes. (Note: polenta can be purchased at health food stores already prepared.)

Succotash

4 cups dry lima or kidney beans (*See Rules for Meal Preparation, Bean Preparation*)
2 cups whole-kernel corn
1 1/2 cups water
1/2 cup combination of red and green peppers, chopped

Combine all the ingredients in a large saucepan in water or a vegetable broth. Cook over low to medium heat, stirring the vegetables. Add the optional chopped sweet red and green pepper. Serves 4 to 6.

Sweet Potato Fries

4 large sweet potatoes, cut like fries
2 tbsp maple syrup
1 tsp vegetable broth
1 tsp ground cinnamon

Toss cut vegetables, broth, cinnamon in a bowl. Transfer to baking sheet. Bake in a 450 oven for about 50 minutes, or until the vegetables are tender. During the last 30 minutes of roasting, toss vegetables occasionally. At the end of baking, toss with maple syrup.

Vegetable Korma

14 fl oz can coconut milk (or fresh coconut milk)
2 oz flaked almonds
1 lb mixed vegetables cut into bite size chunks (e.g., carrot, potato, broccoli, cauliflower, peas)
1 onion, finely chopped
1 tbsp vegetable broth
1 tbsp curry paste

Heat the broth in a large saucepan and cook the onion over a fairly high heat for 5 minutes until golden brown. Stir in the curry paste and cook for 1 minute. Add the vegetables and coconut milk, cover and simmer for 15 minutes until the vegetables are tender. Place the almonds in a frying pan and dry fry for 2-3 minutes, tossing the almonds until golden brown. Season curry to taste with pepper and sprinkle over the toasted almonds. Serve immediately with rice, naan or bread.

Vegetables with Thai Peanut Sauce
Serves 5 to 8

Thai Peanut Sauce
4 cups vegetables, fruits, and nuts
2 tbsp vegetable broth
1 tbsp water
1 tbsp minced garlic

Use any combination of broccoli, carrots, cauliflower, red cabbage, green peppers, scallions, tomatoes, mushrooms, unsalted cashew halves, cilantro, raisins, and pineapple chunks totaling 4 cups. Sauté the vegetable/fruit/nut mixture with the water, garlic, and vegetable broth. Serve over rice topped with Peanut Sauce.

Dinner

Basmati, Vegetables & Fruit
Serves 4

3 cups pineapple chunks
2 unripe bananas
1 medium onion, cubed
1 medium carrot, grated
2 cups broccoli florets
1 cup basmati rice
2 tbsp vegetable broth
1 tbsp chopped parsley
1 tbsp chopped chives
1 tbsp chopped fresh basil
1/2 tsp curry powder

Cook the rice in 2 cups of water for 20 minutes, or until done. Cut the broccoli florets into small flowers. Cut the pineapple into bite-sized pieces and the banana into large slices. Heat the broth in a pan, and add the onion. Add the broccoli and carrot. Lower the heat, cover the pan and let it simmer for a few minutes. Add the curry, pineapple, banana and pepper, and fry for a few more minutes. The vegetables should be just tender. Add the herbs shortly before serving. Serve on rice.

Basmati and Wild Rice Pilaf
Makes about 6 cups

2 garlic cloves, minced
2 stalks celery, thinly sliced
1 onion, finely chopped
2-1/2 cups vegetable broth
2 cups thinly sliced mushrooms
1/2 cup wild rice, rinsed
1/2 cup brown basmati rice, rinsed
1/3 cup chopped pecans
1/3 cup finely chopped parsley
1/2 tsp thyme
1/2 tsp marjoram
1/4 tsp black pepper

Combine wild rice and vegetable broth in a saucepan. Cover and simmer 20 minutes. Add basmati rice, then cover and continue cooking over very low heat until tender, about 50 minutes. Preheat oven to 375. Place pecans in a small oven-proof dish and bake until fragrant, about 8 minutes. Set aside. Heat 1/2 cup of water in a large skillet and cook onion and garlic until all the water has evaporated. Add 1/4 cup of water and cook until the water has evaporated. Repeat until onions are browned, about 20 minutes. Lower heat slightly and add mushrooms, celery, parsley, thyme, marjoram and black pepper. Cook, stirring frequently, for 5 minutes. Add cooked rice and toasted pecans. Stir to mix, then transfer to a baking dish and bake 20 minutes.

Broccoli with Buckwheat and Black Bean Sauce
Makes about 8 cups

2 cups dry black beans (*See Rules for Meal Preparation, Bean Preparation*)
1 large bunch broccoli
4 cups boiling water
2 cups buckwheat groats (or kasha for stronger flavor)
1/2 cup roasted red pepper
2 tbsp lemon juice
2 tbsp vegetable broth
1/2 tsp chili powder
1/4 tsp ground cumin
1/4 tsp ground coriander
1/4 cup chopped fresh cilantro

Cut off broccoli stems. Cut or break the tops into bite-sized florets. Peel the stem with a sharp knife, then slice into 1/2-inch thick rounds. Set aside. Into the water in a large saucepan, place buckwheat groats. Cover and simmer for about 10 minutes, or until all the liquid has been absorbed. While buckwheat (kasha) is cooking, combine and purée all the remaining ingredients in a food processor or blender. Just before you are ready to eat, steam broccoli over boiling water for about 5 minutes, or until it is bright green and just tender. Place a generous about of buckwheat on each serving plate, then top with steamed broccoli and black-bean sauce.

Buckwheat (roasted) Pilaf
Serves 4

1 small carrot, sliced
1 small onion, cut in 8 pieces
1/2 celery rib, sliced
2 cups vegetable broth
1/2 cup whole buckwheat groats (aka kasha)

In a food processor, pulse the carrot, onion and celery until they are finely chopped. In a large, heavy saucepan or small Dutch oven, heat the 2 tablespoons of broth over medium-high heat. Stir in the chopped vegetables. Sauté until they are soft, 4 minutes, stirring occasionally. Mix the buckwheat into the sautéed vegetables. Stir until it is fragrant and looks slightly darker in color, 1-2 minutes. Pour in the broth. Cover the pot tightly. When the liquid boils, reduce the heat and simmer 10 minutes. Turn off the heat and let the pilaf sit 5 minutes. Fluff the pilaf with a fork.

Bulgur Pilaf (spicy)
Makes about 4 cups

1 medium onion, chopped
2 garlic cloves, minced
1/2 red bell pepper, finely diced
1-3/4 cups boiling water or vegetable stock
1 cup bulgur wheat
2 tbsp vegetable broth
2 tsp chili powder
3/4 tsp cumin
1/8 tsp celery seed

Heat broth in a large skillet or pot and cook onion for 3 minutes. Stir in garlic, bulgur, chili powder, cumin, and celery seed. Continue cooking, stirring often, until onion is soft, about 5 minutes. Add bell pepper and boiling water. Stir to mix, then cover and simmer until bulgur is tender and all liquid is absorbed, about 20 minutes. Oven method: Preheat oven to 350. Prepare as above, except before adding boiling water, transfer bulgur mixture to an ovenproof dish. Add boiling water, cover with foil and bake until bulgur is tender and all liquid is absorbed, about 30 minutes.

Bulgur – Spanish
Serves 8

3-1/2 cups boiling water
2 cups bulgur
2 garlic cloves, minced
4-6 tsp chili powder
2 tsp vegetable broth
1 tsp ground cumin

Place the bulgur in a large bowl and pour the boiling water over it. Cover the bowl and let stand 20 minutes, until the bulgur is tender. Drain off any excess water. In a large skillet, sauté the garlic in vegetable broth (or water). Do not let it brown. With the pan still on the heat, stir in the soaked bulgur and add the chili powder and cumin. Turn with a spatula to mix in the spices and continue cooking until the mixture is very hot.

Burger – Beet
Serves 6

1 cup uncooked oats
1/2 cup cooked oats
1/2 cup coarsely ground walnuts
1/4 cup coarsely ground almonds
1/4 cup minced green pepper
1/4 cup minced onion
2 tbsp low-sodium Tamari (soy sauce)
2 tbsp sesame seeds
1 tbsp instant dry vegetable broth
1 tbsp nutritional yeast flakes (optional)
1 tbsp fincly grated raw beet
1 tsp dried basil
1/4 tsp dried thyme
1/4 tsp ground sage
1/4 tsp mustard powder
tomato slices, for garnish

Mix all ingredients together well. Form into 6 patties and grill until cooked through. Serve on whole wheat rolls with tomato slices and your favorite condiments.

Burger – Lentil
Makes 8 burgers

1 small onion, chopped
1/2 cup short-grain brown rice
1/2 cup lentils
2 cups water
1 small carrot
1 medium-sized celery stalk
2 tsp stone-ground mustard
1 tsp garlic powder
Vegetable oil substitute, for skillet

In a medium-sized saucepan, combine onion, rice, lentils, and water. Bring to a slow simmer, then cover and cook for about 50 minutes, or until rice and lentils are tender and all the water has been absorbed. Chop carrot and celery until fine (a food processor makes this easy). Add them to the hot lentil mixture, along with the remaining ingredients. Stir to mix, then chill completely. (You can make the patties while the mixture is still warm, but forming is much easier once it is chilled.) Form mixture into 2- to 3-inch patties. Lightly coat a large skillet with a vegetable oil substitute (e.g., pureed bananas). Cook patties over medium heat for about 4 minutes per side, or until lightly browned.

Burger – Nut and Seed
Makes 4 burgers

1 carrot, grated
1 stalk celery, finely chopped
1/2 cup ground almonds
1/2 cup ground raw sunflower seeds
1/2 cup finely chopped onion
egg replacer equivalent to 1 egg
1 tbsp vegetable broth
1 tsp dill weed
1 tsp marjoram
garlic powder to taste
black pepper to taste

Preheat oven to 350. Grind the nuts in a coffee grinder or food processor, and chop vegetables into small pieces. Mix all the ingredients together, and shape into burgers. Bake for 15 minutes on each side on a cookie sheet.

Chili – Black Bean
Makes 6 cups

4 cups dry black beans (*See Rules for Meal Preparation, Bean Preparation*)
1 4-ounce can diced chilies
2 medium-sized cloves garlic, minced
1 medium-sized onion, chopped
1 small bell pepper, diced fine
1/2 cup water
1/2 cup crushed tomatoes or tomato sauce
1 tsp ground cumin

In a large skillet or pot, heat the water. Add onion, garlic, and pepper. Cook over high heat until onion is translucent. Add remaining ingredients and simmer for about 15 minutes or until flavors are blended.

Chili – Three Bean

(*See Rules for Meal Preparation, Bean Preparation*)
4 cups tomatoes, diced
2 cups dry white beans
2 cups dry black beans
2 cups dry red beans
1 1/2 cup tomato sauce
1 1/2 cups chopped onion
2 tbsp maple syrup
2 tbsp minced garlic
1 tbsp chili powder
2 tsp ground cumin
2 tsp vegetable broth
1 tsp black pepper

Heat broth in large pot over medium-high heat. Cook onions until soft. Drain and rinse three beans and add to onions. Stir in all remaining ingredients. Bring to a boil and then reduce heat to low and simmer for 30 to 45 minutes.

Chili – Vegetarian
Serves 4

4 cups dry pinto beans (*See Rules for Meal Preparation, Bean Preparation*)
1-3 jalapeno peppers, seeded and minced
1 medium yellow onion, chopped
1 medium green bell pepper, cut in ½-inch pieces
1 cup coarsely chopped tomatoes
2 cups vegetable broth, divided
1/4 cup chopped cilantro leaves
2 tsp ground ancho chile, or 1 Tbs. chili powder
1 tbsp finely chopped garlic
1 tsp ground cumin
1 tsp dried oregano
2 tsp masa or corn meal
Freshly ground black pepper, optional

In a medium Dutch oven, sauté the onion, bell pepper and garlic in a small amount of vegetable broth until the onion is translucent.. Add the jalapeno pepper, cumin, ancho chile or chili powder and oregano. Stir until the spices are fragrant. Add the beans, chopped tomatoes, all but 3 tablespoons of the vegetable broth and the cilantro. Set the remaining vegetable broth aside. Bring the chili to a boil. Reduce the heat and simmer, uncovered, for 10 minutes. Place the masa or corn meal in a small bowl. Mix in the reserved vegetable broth, stirring to make a smooth mixture. While stirring the chili, blend in the corn mixture, blending it in well. Add pepper, if desired. Continue simmering the chili 10 minutes longer. For the best flavor, let the chili sit 1-2 hours in the refrigerator. Reheat and serve.

Couscous – Moroccan
Serves 4

1 15-oz. can chick peas
1 sweet potato or small winter squash, cubed
1 zucchini, cubed
1 red bell pepper, diced
1 yellow bell pepper, diced
1 clove garlic, minced or pressed
2 cups uncooked couscous
1/2 cup raisins
1/4 cup water
2 tbsp vegetable broth
1 tsp ground cumin
1/2 tsp allspice
1/2 tsp ground ginger
1/2 tsp turmeric
1/2 tsp paprika
1/4 tsp cayenne
1/4 tsp cinnamon

Sauté the zucchini, sweet potato or squash, and garlic in the broth until partially cooked, about 5 minutes. Use water as necessary to keep the vegetables from sticking. Drain and rinse the chick peas. Add the spices, chick peas, and pepper to the pan. Cover and cook for about 5 minutes. Meanwhile, place the couscous and raisins in another saucepan. Add enough water so that the couscous is covered by about 1/2 inch. Bring the mixture to a boil, then cover tightly, remove from the heat, and let set for at least 10 minutes. Remove the cover from the pepper/chick pea mixture, stir, and cook a few minutes longer to heat thoroughly and thicken.

Curried – Mushrooms, Avocados & Rice

Cooked rice
4 avocadoes
2 tomatoes
1 lb mushrooms
1 large onion
2 tbsp vegetable broth
2 tsp (or more to taste) curry powder
4 tsp lemon juice

Chop the onion. Sauté in the broth along with the mushrooms until tender. Stir in the curry powder and cook for a few moments longer. Chop the tomato and add to the saucepan. Heat through. Add the lemon juice. Stir well and heat until just below boiling point. Peel and halve the avocados. Place on the rice and fill with the mushroom mixture.

Eggplant "Steaks"
Makes 4 servings

2 small eggplants
1 clove garlic, minced
1 tbsp balsamic vinegar
6 tbsp vegetable broth
1 tsp minced fresh parsley
1/2 tsp hot sauce
1/3 tsp dried rosemary

Remove the stem ends from the eggplants and cut off enough of the skin to square the sides. Slice each eggplant lengthwise into two pieces, each approximately 1/2-inch thick. Heat the oven to 350. In a small bowl, stir together 2 tablespoons of broth and the hot sauce. Brush evenly over both sides of the eggplant slices. Bake on a baking sheet for 15 minutes, turning over once. Then broil for 1 minute per side or until the slices are well browned and tender. In a small bowl, stir together the remaining broth, garlic, vinegar, parsley, and rosemary. Brush on the cooked eggplant. Let stand for 5 minutes before serving.

Falafel

2 15oz cans chickpeas
6 scallions, minced
4 cloves garlic, minced
1/3 cup whole wheat flour (or brown rice flour, quinoa flour)
1/4 cup minced fresh parsley
1/4 cup water or reserved bean liquid
1 tbsp lemon juice
1 tsp turmeric
cayenne to taste

Mix everything but flour in food processor (or mash it). Add flour and stir till well mixed. Form into small patties.
Bake at 375, turn, until both sides are crispy. Wrap in spinach leaves. Dip in favorite dressing.

Falafel – Quick
Makes 12 falafels

1 package falafel mix
2 green onions, sliced
6 pieces whole wheat pita bread
4 cups shredded lettuce
1 cup sliced cucumber
1 medium tomato, diced

Prepare falafel patties according to package directions. Warm pocket bread until it is soft. Cut warm pita bread in half and carefully open the pocket. Fill it with two falafel patties. Garnish with lettuce, cucumber, tomato, green onions, and mustard. Repeat with remaining pita bread.

Ginger Noodles
Serves 6 to 8

1 package whole wheat soba noodles (approximately 8 ounces)
2 garlic cloves, minced
2 green onions, finely chopped, including tops
1/4 cup fresh cilantro (optional)
1 jalapeno pepper, finely chopped
3 tbsp seasoned rice vinegar
3 tbsp low-sodium Tamari (soy sauce)
2 tsp finely chopped fresh ginger

Cook the noodles in boiling water according to the package directions. When tender, drain, and rinse. Mix all the remaining ingredients, then pour over the noodles and toss to mix.

Greens and Beans With Garlic
Serves 4

2 cups dry cannellini beans (*See Rules for Meal Preparation, Bean Preparation*)
2 large cloves garlic, minced
3 cups chopped kale
3 cups chopped broccoli rabe
2 cups collards, cut in 1/2-inch ribbons
3 cups fresh spinach or a 10 oz. frozen package, defrosted
1 cup vegetable broth
3/4 cup small leek, white part only, sliced
1/2 cup scallions, green and white parts, chopped
Season to taste.

In a large, heavy skillet over medium heat, sauté the leeks, scallions and garlic in a few tbsp of vegetable broth. Add the kale, broccoli rabe and collards, stirring until they are wilted. Mix in spinach and beans. Add the vegetable broth and simmer until the greens are tender, stirring occasionally. Season to taste. Serve over pasta or polenta.

Mushrooms – Portabello Grilled
Serves 4

4 large portabello mushrooms
2 medium-size cloves garlic, minced
4 tsp of vegetable broth
2 tbsp of red wine
2 tbsp low-sodium Tamari (soy sauce)
1 tbsp of balsamic vinegar

Clean mushrooms and trim stems flush with the bottom of the caps. In a large skillet, mix the remaining ingredients. Heat until the mixture begins to bubble; add mushrooms, tops down. Reduce to medium heat. Cover and cook for about 3 minutes, or until tops are browned. (If pan becomes dry, add 2 to 3 tbsp of water.) Turn the mushrooms and cook for about 5 minutes more, or until tender when pierced with a sharp knife.

Pasta – Artichoke
Makes 4 servings

1 (14-oz.) can artichoke hearts, quartered
1 (12-oz.) can diced tomatoes
2 cups tomatoes, diced
1/2 pound tri-colored whole wheat pasta
2 cloves garlic, minced
1/2 medium onion, chopped
2 tbsp vegetable broth

Cook the pasta according to the package directions. While the pasta is cooking, sauté the onion and garlic in the broth for 1 to 2 minutes. Add the artichokes, tomatoes, and tomato sauce. Drain the pasta and combine all the ingredients.

Pasta – Asparagus
Serves 4

2 pounds fresh asparagus
2 1/2 cups tomatoes, chopped
8 ounces spaghetti
1 medium onion, chopped
2 tbsp water or vegetable stock
1 tbsp chopped fresh basil
1/4 tsp ground sage

Heat water or vegetable stock in a large, pan. Add onion and sauté over medium heat for 3 minutes, until translucent. Add tomatoes, asparagus, basil, and sage. Bring to a boil, cover, and simmer for 7 minutes. Remove from heat and keep warm. Cook pasta in water only without salt. Drain pasta and place in a serving bowl. Add the asparagus mixture and toss.

Pasta – Buckwheat Pasta
Serves 6

12 ounces whole wheat soba noodles
1 medium onion, chopped
3 cups sliced fresh mushrooms
1-1/2 cups cold water
4 tbsp vegetable broth
2 tbsp whole wheat flour
2 tsp low-sodium Tamari (soy sauce)
1/2 tsp garlic powder
1/4 tsp black pepper

Sauté the onion in a large skillet with the broth until transparent, then add the mushrooms. Cover and continue cooking until mushrooms are brown. Whisk flour and water together until smooth, then add to the skillet along with the Tamari, garlic powder, and pepper. Cook, uncovered, over medium-low heat until thickened. Bring water to boil in a large kettle. Add the noodles and boil until al dente, about 8 minutes.

Pasta – Cold Linguine & Asparagus
Makes 4 servings

3/4 lb. asparagus, cut diagonally into 1 1/2-inch pieces
8 oz. linguine whole wheat pasta
1/2 cup orange juice (unsweetened)
1/2 cup sliced green onions (green part only)
2 tbsp low-sodium Tamari (soy sauce)
3 tsp vegetable broth
1 tsp minced roasted garlic
1 tsp grated, fresh ginger root
1 tsp grated orange peel
1/4 tsp brown sugar
Dash hot pepper sauce, or to taste

Cook the noodles according to the package directions. Place the asparagus in a colander. Pour the noodles into the colander, on top of the asparagus, and drain—the hot water and noodles will lightly steam the asparagus. Leave in the colander for 10 minutes. Combine the remaining ingredients in a large bowl and mix well. Add the noodles and asparagus and stir gently until well blended. Refrigerate for several hours or overnight, stirring occasionally. Stir again before serving and serve cold.

Pasta – Lentils and Artichoke Hearts

1 pound farfalle, rotini or other whole wheat pasta
1 1/2 cups artichoke hearts
2 large garlic cloves, pressed or minced
1 bay leaf
1 cup dry red lentils
3 cups water
2 cups tomatoes, coarsely chopped
2 cups diced onions
2 tbsp lemon juice
2 tsp ground cumin
1 tsp ground coriander
1/4 tsp crushed red pepper

Combine the water, lentils, and bay leaf, bring to a boil, lower the heat and simmer for 15-20 min. Sauté onions until golden, add the garlic, cumin, and coriander, stir frequently. Add the lemon juice, tomatoes, artichoke hearts and crushed red pepper and simmer for 10 minutes. Drain the cooked lentils, save some of the cooking liquid (in case sauce is dry). Then add lentils to the tomato mixture, simmer for 10 minutes, adding 1/2 cup of the cooking liquid from lentils if sauce is dry. Boil water for pasta, and then top the pasta with the sauce.

Pasta – Mediterranean

12 or more kalamata olives
4 spring onions, sliced
2 sweet red peppers, sliced thinly
2 cloves of garlic, minced
3 tbsp vegetable broth
Fettuccini, linguini or angel hair

Over a medium flame, sauté the garlic in the broth for a minute. Add the green onions and sauté 2 more minutes. Add the olives and peppers and sauté a few more minutes then take it off heat and serve it over the pasta.

Pasta – Penne with Fresh Spinach, Tomatoes, and Olives
Serves 4

3 cups tomatoes, diced
8 ounces whole wheat penne pasta
1 pound fresh spinach, coarsely chopped
1 medium onion, chopped
1/2 cup kalamata olives, pitted, sliced
2 tbsp vegetable broth
1 tbsp chopped fresh parsley

Heat broth in a large skillet. Add onion and sauté over medium heat for 3 minutes. Add chopped tomatoes. Bring to a boil and then reduce heat, cover, and simmer for 20 minutes. Add sliced olives, chopped spinach, and parsley. Cook an additional 5 minutes. Meanwhile, cook pasta. Drain and transfer to a serving bowl. Add spinach mixture and toss.

Pasta – Roasted Vegetables
Serves 6

16-ounces penne or other bite-sized pasta
10-12 baby bella or cremini mushrooms, quartered
2 Roma tomatoes, chopped
1 medium zucchini, quartered and sliced
1 sweet red pepper, cut into bite-sized chunks
1 small onion, cut into bite-sized chunks
1/2 large eggplant, cut into bite-sized chunks
1/2 head garlic (about 6 cloves)
2 tbsp vegetable broth
2 tsp fresh thyme
crushed red pepper, to taste (optional)

Heat oven to 400. Peel garlic cloves and cut in half. Spread eggplant, zucchini, red pepper, onion, mushrooms, and garlic cloves on a flat pan (baking dish or cookie sheet). Sprinkle with 1 tablespoon of vegetable broth and toss. Roast for 25 to 35 minutes, turning vegetables once during cooking, until vegetables are soft and have crispy edges. Cook pasta according to package directions, drain, and rinse. Toss pasta with vegetables, tomatoes, fresh thyme, and the remaining tablespoon of broth. Serve warm or at room temperature.

Pasta Supper
Makes about 6 cups

2 cups red kidney beans (*See Rules for Meal Preparation, Bean Preparation*)
8 ounces whole wheat pasta spirals
1 onion chopped
2 cups finely chopped fresh kale
1 cup tomato juice
1/2 cup chopped fresh basil
1/4 cup chopped garlic
1 tbsp vegetable broth

Cook the pasta until just tender. Transfer to a colander. Rinse and drain. Set aside. Heat the broth in a large skillet or pot. Add the onion and garlic and cook over medium heat, stirring often. Stir in 1/4 cup of water. Add the tomato juice, kidney beans with their liquid, kale and basil. Stir to mix, then cover and simmer until the kale is tender. Stir in the cooked pasta.

Pie – Tamale

2 cups dry kidney beans (*See Rules for Meal Preparation, Bean Preparation*)
1 1/2 cups fresh or frozen corn kernels
1 can sliced or whole black olives
1 chopped onion
1 chopped bell pepper
1 1/2 pints tomatoes
1 cup cornmeal
1/2 cup water
1 tbsp chili powder
Garlic powder

Mix all together and pour into casserole. Bake at 350, covered, for 30 min. Uncover to brown top.

Pizza
Makes 4 servings.

4 individual whole wheat pizza shells
1 small eggplant, sliced
1 medium zucchini, sliced
1 red onion, cut into small wedges
1 red bell pepper, thinly sliced
1 yellow bell pepper, thinly sliced
2 tbsp vegetable broth
1 tbsp balsamic vinegar
1/2 tsp dried thyme
1/2 tsp black pepper
1/2 cup tomato sauce

Preheat the oven to 425. Combine the eggplant, zucchini, onion, bell peppers, broth, vinegar, thyme, and pepper in a large baking dish and toss to mix well. Bake, stirring occasionally, for 20 minutes, or until the vegetables are tender. Set aside. Place the pizza shells on baking sheets. Spread about 2 tablespoons of the tomato sauce on each pizza shell, then top with the roasted vegetables. Bake for 10 to 12 minutes or until the pizza shells and vegetables are heated through.

Pizza – Pita Pizzas
Makes 6 pizzas

6 pieces of whole wheat pita bread
1 1/2 cup tomato sauce
1 6-ounce can tomato paste
2 green onions, thinly sliced
1 red bell pepper, diced
1 cup chopped mushrooms
1 tsp garlic granules or powder
1/2 tsp basil
1/2 tsp oregano
1/2 tsp thyme

Preheat oven to 375. Combine tomato sauce, tomato paste, garlic granules and herbs. Prepare vegetables as directed. Turn a piece of pita bread upside down and spread with 2 to 3 tablespoons of sauce. Top with chopped vegetables. Repeat with remaining pita breads. Arrange on a baking sheet and bake until edges are lightly browned, about 10 minutes. (Note: Refrigerate or freeze the remaining sauce for use at another time or use with another meal.)

Polenta – Grilled with Portabella Mushrooms
Serves 4

4 large portabella mushrooms
1 roasted red pepper, cut into thin strips for garnish (optional)
2 cups vegetable broth
1/2 cup polenta (coarsely ground cornmeal)
1/2 cup water
2 tbsp vegetable broth
2 tbsp low-sodium Tamari (soy sauce)
2 tbsp balsamic vinegar
2 tbsp red wine
2 garlic cloves, crushed

Combine the polenta, 2 cups vegetable broth, and the 1/2 cup of water in a saucepan. Bring to a simmer and cook, stirring frequently, until very thick, 15 to 20 minutes. Pour into a 9- x 9-inch baking dish and chill completely. To grill, cut into wedges and cook over medium heat until nicely browned. Clean the mushrooms, remove stems. Prepare the marinade by stirring the remaining ingredients together in a large bowl. Place the mushrooms upside down in the marinade and let stand 10 to 15 minutes. Turn right side up and grill over medium-hot coals about 5 minutes. Turn and pour some of the marinade into each of the cavities. Grill until mushrooms can be pierced with a skewer, about 5 minutes longer. Serve with grilled polenta. Garnish with roasted red pepper strips, if desired.

Polenta – Stuffed Peppers
Makes 4 servings.

1 (1-lb.) package cooked polenta
2 medium tomatoes, diced
1 green, 1 red, 1 yellow, and 1 orange bell pepper (or any combination you choose)
2 tbsp vegetable broth
1/2 tsp minced fresh garlic
1/4 tsp pepper
Paprika

Preheat the oven to 375. Cut the tops off the peppers and scoop out the insides. Place peppers on a baking tray. Sauté the garlic in the broth over low heat. Add the tomatoes and pepper. Heat briefly and stir into the polenta.
Fill the peppers with the polenta mixture and sprinkle with paprika. Cook for 30 to 40 minutes.

Potato Pancakes
Serves 4

4 large potatoes, grated
2 carrots, grated
1 medium onion, grated
1/4 cup chopped cilantro
2 tbsp whole wheat flour (optional)

Mix ingredients, press firmly into patties, and cook in pan, pressing down occasionally while cooking. Turn and cook on other side. Serve two pancakes per person, with apple sauce.

Potatoes – Cottage Fries
Serves 6

4 medium red potatoes
1 medium onion, chopped
1 green bell pepper, diced
2 tbsp vegetable broth
1 tsp paprika
1/4 tsp black pepper

Dice potatoes into generous bite-size pieces. Steam over boiling water until they are just tender when pierced with a fork, about 15 minutes. In a large skillet, sauté the onion and bell pepper in 1 teaspoon vegetable broth until the onion is soft, about 5 minutes. Transfer to a bowl and set aside. Add 1 tablespoon broth to the skillet and sauté the potatoes over medium-heat until hot and lightly browned, about 5 minutes. Return the onion mixture to the pan, add remaining ingredients, toss to mix, and serve. Add more broth as needed.

Potatoes – Golden
Serves 6

4 large red potatoes
2 tsp whole mustard seed
1 onion, chopped
1 cup water
1/2 tsp turmeric
1/2 tsp cumin
1/4 tsp ginger
1/8 tsp cayenne
1/8 black pepper
1-1/2 tsp low-sodium Tamari (soy sauce)

Steam potatoes over boiling water until tender when pierced with a fork, 40 to 50 minutes. Cool completely, then cut them into 1/2-inch cubes. Toast the spices in a large skillet for 1 to 2 minutes, then carefully pour in 1/2 cup of the water. Add the chopped onion and cook, stirring frequently, until the onion is soft and most of the liquid has evaporated, about 5 minutes. Add the potatoes along with the remaining water and the Tamari. Stir to mix, then cover and cook over medium heat for 5 minutes. Stir before serving.

Quesadillas
Makes 8 quesadillas

2 cups dry garbanzo beans (*See Rules for Meal Preparation, Bean Preparation*)
8 corn tortillas
1 garlic clove, peeled
1/2 cup chopped green onions
1/2 cup salsa
1/2 cup water-packed, roasted red pepper
3 tbsp lemon juice
1 tbsp vegetable broth
1/4 tsp cumin

Drain garbanzo beans and place in a food processor or blender with roasted peppers, lemon juice, broth, garlic, and cumin. Process until very smooth, 1 to 2 minutes. Spread a tortilla with 2 to 3 tablespoons of garbanzo mixture and place in a large skillet over medium heat. Sprinkle with chopped green onions, and salsa. Top with a second tortilla and cook until the bottom tortilla is warm and soft, 2-3 minutes. Turn and cook the second side for another minute. Remove from pan and cut in half. Repeat with remaining tortillas.

Ratatouille
Makes 4 to 5 servings.

4-5 cloves garlic, crushed
2 large tomatoes, cut into medium wedges
1 medium zucchini, sliced
1 green bell pepper, chopped
1 red bell pepper, chopped
1 small eggplant, cut into small cubes
1 large onion, diced
1 bay leaf
1/2 cup tomato juice
5 tbsp tomato paste
4 tbsp dry red wine
1 tbsp vegetable broth
1 tbsp dried basil
1/2 tbsp dried marjoram
1/2 tbsp dried oregano
1/2 tsp black pepper
Dash of ground rosemary

Sauté the onion in the broth until translucent. Add the bay leaf and tomato juice and stir well. Then add the garlic, herbs and pepper and mix until well blended. Cover the saucepan and simmer for 10 minutes over low heat. Add the zucchini and peppers, stir well, cover, and simmer for another 5 minutes. Add the eggplant, tomatoes, and tomato paste and stir again. Cover and continue to simmer until the vegetables are tender, about 8 minutes more. Serve over rice or with crusty French bread.

Rotini with Ginger Peanut Sauce
Serves 6

8 ounces rotini
2 tbsp peanut butter
1 to 2 tbsp chopped fresh ginger root
1 tbsp low-sodium Tamari (soy sauce)
1-1/2 tbsp vinegar
1 tsp Dijon mustard
1 cup steamed carrots
1 cup steamed broccoli
3 scallions, finely chopped

Boil the rotini until tender. Drain, saving 1/2 cup of the water. In a blender, whir the 1/2-cup pasta water and the ginger, peanut butter, Tamari, vinegar, and mustard. Toss pasta with sauce. Top with carrots, broccoli, and chopped scallions. (Note: you can use prepared peanut sauce instead of making it.)

Sandwich – Chickpea Pita Pockets

4 whole wheat pitas
1 16 oz can chick peas, rinsed, drained and mashed
1/3 cup chopped celery
1 t minced onion
2 t pickle relish (or piccalilly)
2 t mustard
Dash of garlic powder
Lettuce, tomato slices, grated carrot, etc for toppings

Place the chickpeas, celery, onion, relish, mustard and garlic powder in a bowl and mix well. Cut the pitas in half and open up into pockets. Fill each pita pocket with 1/4 of the chickpea spread, top with lettuce, tomato or other vegetables and serve.

Sandwich – Garbanzo Salad
Makes 4 sandwiches

2 cups dry garbanzo beans (*See Rules for Meal Preparation, Bean Preparation*)
8 slices whole wheat bread
4 lettuce leaves
4 tomato slices
1 stalk celery, finely sliced
1 green onion, finely chopped
1 tbsp sweet pickle relish

Mash garbanzo beans with a fork or potato masher, leaving some chunks. Add sliced celery, chopped onion and pickle relish. Spread on whole wheat bread and top with lettuce and sliced tomatoes.

Sandwich – Grilled Portobello
Serves 4

4 large Portobello mushrooms
4 whole wheat buns
1 cup red wine vinegar
1 cup vegetable broth
1 cup low-sodium Tamari (soy sauce)
Grilled onion

Take equal parts of red wine vinegar, vegetable broth and Tamari and place in a blender to mix then pour over the mushrooms. Let them sit overnight then grill. Add onion and other toppings and a bun.

Sandwich – Toasted Wheat Roll

Whole wheat sandwich roll
Lettuce
Tomato
Onions
Pickles
Pepperoncini (Tuscan peppers)
Basil
Pepper
Dijon Mustard
Slice ingredients so they all fit onto a sandwich roll. Toast bun. Add mustard and any other seasoning or sauce.

Spinach with Garlic
Serves 4

1 large bunch of fresh spinach
3 cloves of garlic
1 tsp vegetarian Worcestershire sauce

Wash and de-stem spinach. Peel and mince garlic. Braise garlic in Worcestershire sauce over medium heat, stirring, until lightly browned. Add spinach to hot skillet. Use tongs to turn spinach until it is just wilted. Serve hot or at room temperature.

Squash – Pinto Beans
Makes 4 servings

2 cups dry pinto beans (*See Rules for Meal Preparation, Bean Preparation*)
1 cup diced tomatoes
2 garlic cloves, minced
3 thyme sprigs
2 cups hot cooked brown rice
1 cup (1/2-inch-thick) sliced yellow squash
1 cup (1/2-inch-thick) sliced zucchini
1/2 cup fresh corn kernels
1/2 cup chopped onion
1/4 cup vegetable broth (or more, as needed, to sauté in)
2 tsp minced seeded jalapeno pepper

Heat broth in a large skillet over medium-high heat. Add the onion, jalapeno, and garlic, and sauté 2 minutes. Stir in squash and zucchini, and sauté 2 minutes. Add corn, beans, tomatoes, and thyme; cover, reduce heat, and simmer 10 minutes. Discard thyme. Serve over rice.

Squash – Spanish
Serves 4

1 8-ounce package of button mushrooms, sliced
2 small zucchini, quartered lengthwise and sliced
1 small yellow onion, finely chopped
1-1/2 cups frozen corn
2 tbsp water
1/2 tsp cumin
1/2 tsp chili powder

Braise onion in 1 tablespoon of water, stirring until liquid has evaporated. Add sliced zucchini, mushrooms, and the remaining water. Stir in spices and simmer for 5 minutes, covered, until mushrooms are soft. Stir in corn and cook for 2 more minutes to heat through. Add black pepper to taste.

Squash – Winter
Makes 4 cups

1 medium winter squash (e.g., butternut)
1/2 cup water
2 tsp low-sodium Tamari (soy sauce)
2 tbsp maple syrup

Slice the squash in half and then peel and remove the seeds. Cut the squash into 1-inch cubes. Place cubes into a large pot with the water. Add the Tamari and syrup. Cover and simmer over medium heat for 15 to 20 minutes, or until squash is tender when pierced with a fork.

Split Pea – Indian Dahl
Serves 6

1 large onion, chopped
1 small green pepper, chopped
1-1/2 cups yellow split peas
3 cups water
1/2 cup water
1-1/2 tsp black mustard seeds
1 tsp turmeric
1/2 tsp curry powder
juice of 1 lemon

Simmer split peas in 3 cups water for 30 minutes or until tender. Add more water, if needed. In another saucepan, simmer chopped onions, green peppers, turmeric, curry powder, mustard seeds and 1/2 cup water for 15 minutes or until onions and peppers are tender. Mix with peas and add lemon juice. Serve over a generous portion of brown rice.

Stir Fry – Sesame Bok Choy & Carrot
Serves 2

5 cups bok choy, cut into 1/2-inch pieces
4 cloves garlic, minced
3 carrots, cut diagonally into 1/4-inch slices
3 cups cooked quinoa
1/2 cup chopped green onions
1/4 cup vegetable broth
2 tsp minced ginger root
2 tbsp toasted sesame seeds

In a large skillet or wok, stir-fry garlic, carrots and green onions in 3 tbsp vegetable broth for 3 minutes. Add bok choy and stir-fry another 2 minutes. Stir in vegetable broth and ginger. Reduce heat and simmer 5 minutes. Sprinkle sesame seeds over stir-fry. Spoon over quinoa.

Stir Fry – Vegetables
Makes 4 to 6 servings.

3 carrots, cut into 2-inch strips
2 green onions, chopped
1 medium onion, sliced
1 green pepper, sliced
2 cups cooked rice
1 cup cauliflower florets
1 cup broccoli florets
1 cup snow peas
1 cup sliced mushrooms
1/4 cup low-sodium Tamari (soy sauce)
1/4 cup lemon juice
1/3 cup vegetable broth
1-2 tsp grated fresh ginger root

Mix together the Tamari, lemon juice, and ginger. Heat the broth in a large pan and add the cauliflower, broccoli, carrots, onion, green pepper. Stir frequently, cooking evenly. Add the snow peas, mushrooms, and green onions. Continue to stir frequently until the vegetables are cooked but still crunchy. Serve over rice, topped with the marinade.

Tabouli
Serves 6

4 green onions, chopped
1 cucumber, chopped
1 tomato, chopped
1 red pepper, chopped
1 cup boiling water
1 cup bulgur
1/2 cup parsley, minced

Let soak for 30 minutes bulgur and boiling water or until water is absorbed: Stir in remaining ingredients. Toss well and chill. Add favorite dressing.

Tabouli – Quinoa
Serves 4 to 6

2 small tomatoes
3 green onions, chopped
2-1/2 cups cooked quinoa (1 cup dry)
2 cups finely chopped parsley
3/4 cup chopped mint
1/2 cup diced seedless cucumbers
3 tbsp lemon juice
1 tbsp vegetable broth
1/4 tsp black pepper

Rinse quinoa thoroughly. Bring 1 cup quinoa and 1-3/4 cup water to a full boil over medium heat, cover, and reduce to simmer. Continue simmering for 15 minutes. Remove from heat and uncover. Allow to cool. In a bowl, combine quinoa, mint, cucumbers, parsley, tomatoes, and onions. In a small bowl, whisk together the lemon juice, broth and pepper. Pour over salad; toss. Serve at room temperature or refrigerate and serve cold.

Tacos and More

Brown rice
Cooked black beans (*See Rules for Meal Preparation, Bean Preparation*)
Chopped tomatoes
Chopped videlia, green or any onion
Frozen corn thawed in hot water
Chopped red, yellow or green peppers
Grated or julienned carrots
Water chestnuts
Chopped cilantro
Chopped arugala
Low-sodium Tamari (soy sauce)
Salsa
Taco shells (whole wheat)

Cook rice. Heat beans. Put all chopped vegetables in individual dishes. Start on your plate with rice and just pile it up high and top it all with low-sodium Tamari and/or salsa. Put all leftovers in a bowl and use for salad the next day adding balsamic vinegar.

Vegetables – Grilled
Makes about 4 servings

2 ears fresh corn
1 red onion
1 red bell pepper
1 medium zucchini or other summer squash
2 cups button mushrooms
2 tsp vegetable broth
2 tsp garlic granules or powder
2 tsp mixed Italian herbs
2 tsp chili powder

Preheat grill. Cut onion, bell pepper, and zucchini into generous chunks. Place in a large mixing bowl. Clean mushrooms and add. Husk corn, cut it into 1-inch lengths, and add. Sprinkle vegetables with broth and toss to coat. Sprinkle with garlic granules, Italian herbs and chili powder. Toss to mix. Spread vegetables in a single layer on a grilling rack and place over medium-hot coals. Cover and cook 5 minutes. Turn with a spatula and cook until tender when pierced with a sharp knife, about 5 more minutes. Repeat with remaining vegetables.

Wraps – Thai Wraps
Serves 6

6 large flour tortillas
1 small onion, chopped
1 carrot, thinly sliced
1 celery stalk, thinly sliced
1/2 red bell pepper, diced
2 cups sliced mushrooms
2 cups finely chopped kale
2 cups cooked brown rice
1/2 cup chopped cilantro
6 tbsp Plum Sauce
1 tbsp peanut butter
2 tbsp low-sodium Tamari (soy sauce)
1-1/2 tsp curry powder

Mix the peanut butter with 3 tablespoons of water. Set aside. Heat 1/2 cup of water and the Tamari in a large skillet. Add the onion, carrot, celery, and mushrooms and cook until the vegetables are tender. Stir in the curry powder, red bell pepper, cilantro, kale, and peanut butter mixture. Cover and cook until the kale is tender. Heat the tortillas in a dry skillet until soft. Place about 1/2 cup of the vegetable mixture along the center of the tortilla. Top with 1/4 cup of brown rice and 2 tsp of Plum Sauce. Roll the tortilla around the filling.

Wraps – Veggie Wrap
Makes 4 wraps

4 whole wheat tortillas
1 carrot, shredded
1 cup bean sprouts
1–2 cups hummus
1–2 cups mixed salad greens or torn leaf lettuce
1/4 cup sunflower seeds

Preheat oven or toaster oven to 375. Place sunflower seeds in a small ovenproof dish and roast until lightly browned and fragrant. Set aside. Warm tortillas, one at a time, in a large dry skillet, flipping to warm both sides until soft and pliable. Spread each tortilla evenly with about 1/2 cup of hummus, leaving edges uncovered. Divide remaining ingredients evenly among tortillas. Wrap tortillas around filling.

Yams and Bok Choy
Serves 4

2 large cloves of garlic, minced
2 small bok choy, finely sliced
2 small yams, cut into bite-sized chunks
1 onion, sliced and quartered
1 tbsp vegetarian Worcestershire sauce
1/2 tsp Thai chili paste
1/2 lemon

Put yams in a deep skillet and just cover them with water. Cover skillet and boil yams 5 to 10 minutes until soft when pierced with a fork. Add onions and garlic and continue to simmer until about half of the water has boiled away. Add Worcestershire sauce, chili paste, and bok choy. Simmer until the bok choy is soft. Squeeze lemon over the mixture and serve.

Yams With Cranberries and Apples
Serves 8

4 yams, peeled
1 large, green apple, peeled and diced
1 cup raw cranberries
1/2 cup raisins
1/2 cup organic orange juice
2 tbsp maple syrup
Maple syrup

Preheat oven to 350. Cut peeled yams into 1-inch chunks and place in a large baking dish. Top with diced apple, cranberries, and raisins. Sprinkle with maple syrup or other sweetener, then pour orange juice over all. Cover and bake for 1 hour and 15 minutes, or until yams are tender when pierced with a fork.

Dips, Spreads and Sauces

Apple Chutney
Makes 3 cups

1-1/2 pounds tart apples (about 3 large apples)
1 medium garlic clove, minced
1 cup raw, maple syrup
1 cup cider vinegar
1/2 cup water
1 tbsp chopped fresh ginger or 1/2 tsp ground ginger
1 tsp each ground cinnamon and cloves
1/4 tsp cayenne, or more to taste

Coarsely chop the apples, then combine them with all the remaining ingredients in a heavy saucepan. Bring to a boil, then lower heat and simmer uncovered, stirring occasionally, for 1 hour, until most of the liquid is absorbed.

Balsamic Vinaigrette
Makes 1 cup

1 garlic clove, pressed
2 tbsp balsamic vinegar
2 tbsp seasoned rice vinegar
1 tbsp ketchup
1 tsp stone ground mustard

Whisk all ingredients together.

Bread Dressing
Makes about 4 cups

3 cups sliced mushrooms (about 1/2 pound)
2 celery stalks, thinly sliced
1 onion, chopped
4 cups cubed whole wheat bread
1 cup vegetable broth
1/3 cup finely chopped parsley
1 tbsp vegetable broth
1/2 tsp thyme
1/2 tsp marjoram
1/2 tsp sage
1/8 tsp black pepper

Sauté onion in broth until translucent. Add sliced mushrooms and celery. Cover and cook over medium heat, stirring occasionally, for 5 minutes. Preheat oven to 350. Stir bread into onion mixture, along with parsley, thyme, marjoram, sage, and black pepper. Lower heat and continue cooking 3 minutes, stirring often. Stir in vegetable broth, a little at a time, until dressing obtains desired moistness. Spread in a baking dish, cover and bake 20 minutes. Remove cover and bake 10 minutes longer.

Brown Gravy
Makes 2 cups

2 cups water or vegetable broth
3 tbsp low-sodium Tamari (soy sauce)
2 tbsp cornstarch
1 tbsp cashews
1 tbsp onion powder
1/2 tsp garlic granules or powder

Pour water or broth into a blender. Add cashews, onion powder, garlic granules, cornstarch, and Tamari. Blend until completely smooth, 2 to 3 minutes. Transfer to a saucepan and cook over medium heat, stirring constantly, until thickened.

"Cheese" Sauce

2 cups water
1/2 cup nutritional yeast flakes
1/2 cup whole wheat flour
1/2 tsp garlic powder
1/4 cup vegetable broth
1 tsp wet mustard

In a 2-quart saucepan, mix together nutritional yeast flakes, flour and garlic powder, then 2 cups water. Cook over medium heat, whisking until it thickens and bubbles. Cook 30 seconds more, then remove from head and whisk in vegetable broth and mustard. Sauce will thicken as it cools but will thin when heated. Good for a casserole, as a topping for lasagna, or a pan of enchiladas.

"Cheesy" Garbanzo Spread
Makes about 2 cups

2 cups dry garbanzo beans (*See Rules for Meal Preparation, Bean Preparation*)
1/2 cup roasted red peppers
3 tbsp vegetable broth
3 tbsp lemon juice

Drain the garbanzo beans and place all ingredients in a food processor or blender. Process until very smooth. If using a blender, you will have to stop it occasionally and push everything down into the blades with a rubber spatula. The mixture should be quite thick, but to thin add a tablespoon or two of water.

Chunky Ratatouille Sauce
Serves 6

1 1/2 cups tomatoes, coarsely chopped
8 ounces of cremini mushrooms (also called baby bellas)
6 cloves garlic, minced
2 stalks celery, chopped
2 small onions, chopped
1 large eggplant, cut into 1-inch chunks
1/2 cup vegetable broth
1/4 to 1/2 cup water
1 tsp Italian herbs
1/2 tsp thyme
1/2 tsp black pepper (add more to taste)

Soak eggplant chunks in water for 10 minutes. Drain, rinse, and drain again.
Braise onion, celery, and garlic in 1/4 cup of broth. When the vegetables are soft,
add the eggplant chunks and 1/4 cup of water. Simmer, stirring occasionally,
until the eggplant is soft. Add more water, if necessary, to keep mixture from
drying out. Add mushrooms, spices, remaining wine, and can of tomatoes.
Simmer for 5 minutes. Serve over whole wheat pasta shells, brown rice, or your
favorite grain.

Corn Butter
Makes about 2 cups

1 cup boiling water
1/4 cup cornmeal
2 tbsp raw cashews
1-1/2 tsp agar powder
1 tbsp finely grated carrot
1 tsp nutritional yeast (optional)
2 tsp lemon juice

Combine the cornmeal with 1 cup of water in a small saucepan. Simmer, stirring
frequently, until very thick, about 10 minutes. Set aside. Combine the agar
powder with 1/4 cup of cold water in a blender. Let stand at least 3 minutes. Add
1 cup boiling water and blend to mix. Add the cooked cornmeal, cashews, lemon
juice, grated carrot, and yeast if using. Cover and blend until totally smooth.
Transfer to a covered container and chill until thickened, 2-3 hours.

Cranberry Persimmon Relish
Makes about 2 cups

2 fuyu persimmons
1 cup cranberries, fresh or frozen
2 tbsp orange juice concentrate
1 tbsp maple syrup
1/2 tsp ginger

Remove stems, then coarsely chop persimmons in a food processor. Add cranberries, orange juice concentrate, syrup and ginger. Process using quick pulses until coarsely and uniformly chopped. Let stand 20 minutes before serving.

Creamy Spinach Dip
Serves 10 to 12

1 package frozen spinach, thawed and drained
1 package vegetable soup mix
1 container Tofutti (non-dairy) sour cream
1 tbsp lemon juice
1/2 cup salsa

Combine ingredients and refrigerate for 1 hour before serving. Serve with raw vegetable pieces or chunks of crusty bread.

Garlic Bean Dip
Serves 2

2 cloves garlic, minced
1-1/2 tbsp vegetable broth
1/3 pound green beans
1 tsp low-sodium Tamari (soy sauce)
1/2 tsp onion powder

Steam green beans for 10 minutes in about a cup of water until tender. Rinse beans under cold water when done. Place remaining ingredients in a blender or food processor. Add cooked beans. Blend 2 minutes or until creamy. Serve with whole wheat crackers.

Guacamole
Serves 6

1 avocado
2 cups cooked peas or 1 cup cooked green beans
2 tbsp chopped onion
1/4 cup salsa (or more to taste)
2 tbsp fresh lime juice

Blend the avocado and peas or green beans together in a blender, until smooth. Stir in the onion and salsa. Just before serving, stir in the fresh lime juice.

Hummus Dip
Makes 2 cups

2 cups dry garbanzo beans (*See Rules for Meal Preparation, Bean Preparation*)
1 garlic clove (or more to taste)
2 (or more) tbsp of vegetable broth (add more if needed for consistency)
2 tbsp of lemon juice
1/4 tsp ground cumin.

Put everything in a food processor and let it rip until smooth.

Maple Sweet Potato Spread
Makes about 2 cups

3 dried figs, finely chopped
1 large sweet potato, peeled and quartered
1 small onion, peeled and quartered
1 tbsp vegetable broth
1 tbsp maple syrup

Steam sweet potato and onion pieces until soft. Transfer to a food processor with remaining ingredients. Blend until thick and smooth. Pour into a small container. Keep covered and refrigerate until ready to serve.

Mint Chutney
Makes 1/4 cup

2/3 cup fresh mint leaves
1/4 cup ground walnuts
1 tsp soy sour cream
1/2 tsp tumeric

Wash, dry, and mince the mint leaves. Mix them with the walnuts. In a small cup, stir the soy sour cream and tumeric together, then blend with the mint and walnuts. Cover and allow to set for 30 minutes before serving.

Mustard and Vinegar Dressing
Makes 3/4 cups

2-3 medium cloves
1/2 cup mustard
3 tbsp lemon juice or rice or cider vinegar
3 tbsp water
1 tsp light miso
1 tsp low-sodium Tamari (soy sauce)
1/2 tsp maple syrup
1/2 tsp curry powder

Purée all the ingredients in a blender

Peanut Sauce
Serves 5 to 8

1 cup low-sodium Tamari (soy sauce)
1 cup peanut butter
1/4 cup water
1/4 cup cooking sherry
1 cup lemon or lime juice
2 tbsp minced fresh garlic
1 tbsp red curry paste
1/2 tbsp onion powder
1/2 tbsp basil
1/2 tsp cayenne
1/4 tsp paprika
2 to 3 dashes of Tabasco

Mix all ingredients using a whisk or blender, until creamy.

Plum Sauce

1 17-ounce can purple plums in heavy syrup
2 garlic cloves
2 tbsp seasoned rice vinegar
1 tbsp cornstarch
1 tbsp low-sodium Tamari (soy sauce)
1/8 tsp cayenne (more or less to taste)

Remove pits from the plums, then purée plums in a blender or food processor along with their liquid and the remaining ingredients. Heat in a saucepan, stirring constantly, until thickened.

Refried Beans
Makes about 5 cups

1 1/2 cups dry pinto beans
1 cup crushed or finely chopped tomatoes
1 4-ounce can diced green chilies
1 onion, chopped
4 garlic cloves, minced or pressed
1 1/2 tsp cumin
1/4 tsp cayenne

Clean and rinse beans, then soak in about 6 cups of water for 6 to 8 hours. Discard soaking water, rinse beans and place in a large pot with 4 cups of fresh water, minced garlic, cumin, and cayenne. Simmer until tender, about 1 hour. Heat 1/2 cup of water in a large skillet. Add onion and cook until soft, about 5 minutes. Stir in tomatoes and diced chilies. Cook, uncovered, over medium heat for 10 minutes, stirring occasionally. Add cooked beans, including some cooking liquid, a cup at a time to tomato mixture. Mash some of the beans as you add them. When all the beans have been added, stir to mix, then cook over low heat, stirring frequently, until thickened.

Salsa Fresca
Makes about 6 cups

1 1/2 cups tomato sauce
4 ripe tomatoes, chopped (about 4 cups)
4 garlic cloves, minced
1 small onion, finely chopped
1 bell pepper, finely chopped
1 jalapeño pepper, seeded and finely chopped or 1 teaspoon red pepper flakes (more or less to taste)
1 cup chopped cilantro leaves
2 tbsp cider vinegar
1-1/2 tsp cumin

Combine all ingredients in a mixing bowl. Stir to mix. Let stand 1 hour before serving.

Desserts

Apple Crisp
Serves 10

4 large tart apples
1-1/2 cups rolled oats
3/4 cup natural sweetener
1/2 cup flour
1/3 cup soy or rice margarine
1 tsp cinnamon

Preheat the oven to 350. Peel the apples, if desired, then core and slice them thinly. Toss with 1/2-cup sweetener, 1 tablespoon flour, and cinnamon. Spread evenly in a 9- x 13-inch baking dish. Mix the rolled oats with the remaining flour and sweetener. Add the margarine and work the mixture until it is uniformly crumbly. Sprinkle evenly over the fruit. Bake for 45 minutes, until lightly browned. Let stand 10 minutes before serving.

Applesauce - Strawberry
Makes 2 cups

2 cups peeled, cored, and coarse-chopped apples
2 cups hulled strawberries, fresh or frozen
1/2 cup frozen apple juice concentrate

In a medium-sized saucepan combine all ingredients. Bring to a simmer, then cover and cook over very low heat for about 25 minutes, or until apples are tender. Mash lightly or purée in a food processor, if desired.

Banana Cake
Serves 8

4 ripe bananas
2 cups whole wheat pastry flour
1-1/2 tsp baking soda
1 cup chopped walnuts
1/2 cup maple syrup (or to taste)
1/3 cup applesauce
1/4 cup water
1 tsp vanilla extract

Preheat oven to 350. Mix flour, baking soda in a bowl. In a large bowl, beat maple syrup, applesauce together. Add bananas and mash them. Stir in water and vanilla, mix thoroughly. Add flour mixture, chopped walnuts and stir to mix. Spread in a 9-inch square baking pan. Bake for 45 to 50 minutes, or until a toothpick inserted into the center comes out clean.

Berry Cobbler
One 9 x 9-inch cobbler

Berry mixture:
5-6 cups fresh or frozen berries (blueberries, blackberries, raspberries, or a mixture)
1/4 cup whole wheat pastry flour
1/2 cup natural sweetener

Topping:
1 cup whole wheat pastry flour
2/3 cup water
2 tbsp natural sweetener
1-1/2 tsp baking powder

Preheat oven to 375. Spread berries in a 9 x 9-inch baking dish. Mix in flour and sugar. Place in oven until hot or about 15 minutes. To prepare topping, mix flour, sugar, baking powder in a bowl. Add water and stir until batter is smooth. Spread evenly over hot berries, then bake until golden brown, 25 to 30 minutes.

Berry Sauce
Serves 6 (as dessert topping)

1-1/2 cup frozen raspberries
1 cup fresh or frozen blueberries
1/4 cup orange juice

Combine raspberries and orange juice in a small saucepan. Simmer until raspberries become sauce like, about 5 minutes. Add blueberries and cook for 2 more minutes. Serve warm over fruit sorbet, poached pears, or vanilla non-dairy ice cream.

Fresh Peach Cobbler
Serves 8

4 cups fresh peaches, sliced
1 1/2 cup water
1 cup whole wheat pastry flour
1/2 cup natural sweetener
2 tbsp cornstarch or arrowroot powder
1-1/2 tsp baking powder
ground cinnamon, to taste

Combine 2 tablespoons of natural sweetener and cornstarch in a saucepan, then stir in the peaches and water. Bring to a boil, then boil 1 minute, stirring constantly. Pour into a 9-inch square baking dish, and sprinkle with cinnamon. Preheat oven to 400. Combine flour, 1/2 cup natural sweetener and baking powder. Blend until mixture resembles cornmeal (add water if necessary). Stir in water until mixed, then drop by spoonfuls onto the hot fruit. Bake until golden brown, about 25 minutes.

Gingerbread Cookies
Makes about 48 cookies

2-1/4 cups whole wheat pastry flour
1/3 cup molasses
1/3 cup water
1/2 cup maple syrup
1-1/2 tsp baking soda
1 tsp powdered ginger
1 tsp cinnamon

Mix the maple syrup, ginger, cinnamon and baking soda in a large bowl. Add the molasses and water and mix well. Add 1 cup of flour and mix well. Mix in enough of the remaining flour to make a very stiff dough. Preheat oven to 275. Dust 2-3 baking sheets with flour. On a floured surface, roll a portion of the dough with a flour-dusted rolling pin to a very fine thickness, about 1/16-inch thickness. Cut the dough into shapes with a flour-dusted cookie cutters or a flour-dusted knife. Transfer cookies to the baking sheets. Bake until the edges are dry and the centers give just slightly when pressed, about 20 minutes. Allow to cool on a baking sheet for 5 minutes, then transfer with a spatula to a wire rack to cool. Once cooled, store in an airtight container.

Gingered Melon Wedges
Serves 6

1 large cantaloupe
1 tbsp natural sweetener
1 tbsp candied ginger (optional)
1/2 tsp ground ginger

Cut melon in half and seed. Then cut each half into chunks. Stir together sweetener and ground ginger. Sprinkle over melon chunks and chill.

Fruit Compote

Makes 2 cups

2 cups sliced fresh peaches
2 cups hulled fresh strawberries
1/2 cup white grape juice concentrate or apple juice concentrate

In a large saucepan combine all ingredients. Bring to a simmer and cook for about 5 minutes, or until fruit just becomes soft. Serve warm or cold.

Fruit Gel

Makes about 4 cups

2 cups blueberries, fresh or frozen
1-1/2 cups strawberries, fresh or frozen
3/4 cups apple juice concentrate
1/2 cup water
1/2 tsp agar powder
1 tbsp kudzu powder

Chop strawberries by hand or in a food processor. Transfer to a pan. Add apple juice concentrate, water, agar, and kudzu. Stir to mix. Bring to a simmer and cook 3 minutes, stirring often. Remove from heat and chill completely. Fold in blueberries and transfer to serving dishes.

Monkey Bars
Makes 24 small bars

4 small firm ripe bananas (about 1 pound)
1/2 cup crispy brown rice cereal
1 tbsp natural peanut butter
1 tbsp maple syrup
1 tsp unsweetened cocoa

Cut the bananas in half lengthwise and set aside. Combine all other ingredients in small bowl, blending well. Spread 1 tablespoon of the brown rice/peanut butter mixture over the cut sides of 4 banana halves and then top with the remaining halves. Cut each crosswise into 6 pieces.

Nutty Fruit Balls
Makes about 30 pieces

2/3 cup raisins
2/3 cup golden raisins
2/3 cup dried apricots
2/3 cup dried figs
2/3 cup cashews
1/2 cup peanut butter
1/2 cup carob powder
1/3 cup pitted dates

Grind the dried fruits and nuts into small pieces in a food grinder or heavy-duty food processor. Add the peanut butter and carob powder, mixing thoroughly. Roll into balls the size of walnuts.

Peaches (flambé) with Berries

Fresh or frozen raspberries or blueberries
1 ripe peach
 2 tsp natural sweetener
1 tsp lemon juice

Wash and halve peach. Remove pit. Place peach half, flat side up, in center of a square piece of doubled aluminum foil. Fill cavity of peach half with fresh or frozen raspberries or blueberries. Sprinkle the sweetener and lemon juice on the top. Wrap in foil. Grill approximately 15-20 minutes over hot flame, turning once.

Peanut Butter Balls

Makes 20 balls

3/4 cup peanut butter
1/4 cup low-fat granola
1/4 cup sunflower seeds
1/4 cup raisins
1/4 cup finely shredded carrots
2 tbsp natural sweetener

Mix together the granola, sweetener, sunflower seeds, raisins, and carrots. Blend in the peanut butter a little at a time to form a smooth mixture. Store the mixture in the refrigerator overnight. Form into balls.

Pudding – Brown Rice
Makes about 3 cups

2 cups cooked brown rice
1 1/2 cups water
1/3 cup raisins
1/4 cup maple syrup
1 tbsp cornstarch
1/4 tsp cinnamon
1 tsp vanilla

Whisk water and cornstarch together in a medium saucepan. Add cooked rice, maple syrup, raisins, and cinnamon. Simmer over medium heat 3 minutes, stirring constantly. Remove from heat and stir in vanilla. Serve warm or cold.

Pudding – Chocolate
Makes about 2 cups

2 cups water
1/2 cup natural sweetener
5 tbsp cornstarch
3 tbsp cocoa
1 tsp vanilla

Combine water, cocoa, cornstarch, sugar, and vanilla in a saucepan. Whisk smooth. Cook over medium heat, stirring constantly until pudding is very thick. Pour into individual serving dishes and chill.

Pudding – Fruit
Serves 4

8 to 10 dried apricot halves
2 to 3 medium dried figs
1 medium apple
3 cups water
1 cup quick rolled oats
1/4 cup raisins
1/4 tsp cinnamon

Chop the apricot halves, figs, and raisins in a food processor. Cut and core the apple and then add to fruit in food processor. Chop fine. Transfer the mixture to a medium-sized saucepan and add remaining ingredients. Simmer slowly for about 5 minutes, or until thickened.

Pudding – Sweet Potato
Makes about 1 1/2 cups

1 cup cooked sweet potato or yam
1/2 cup water
1/3 cup rolled oats
1 tbsp maple syrup
1/4 tsp cinnamon

Combine all ingredients in a blender and blend until smooth.

Pudding – Rice
Makes 6 1/2-cup servings

2 cups cooked brown rice
1-1/2 cups water
3 tbsp raisins
2 tbsp maple syrup
1 tsp vanilla extract
1/4 tsp cinnamon
1/4 tsp vanilla extract

In a medium-size saucepan, combine all ingredients and bring to a slow simmer.
Cook uncovered for about 20 minutes, or until thick. Serve hot or cold.

Pudding – Vanilla
Makes about 3 cups

2 cups water
1 cup cooked, peeled yam
5 tbsp maple syrup
2 tbsp cornstarch
1 tbsp potato flour
1/2 tsp vanilla extract

Combine water, cooked yam, and maple syrup in a blender and process until
completely smooth. With blender running, add cornstarch, potato flour and
vanilla extract. Transfer to a saucepan and heat, stirring constantly, until mixture
bubbles and thickens. Remove from heat and transfer to individual serving dishes
if desired. Cool before serving.

Pumpkin Raisin Cookies
Makes 24 3-inch cookies

2 cups whole wheat pastry flour
1 cup pumpkin
1/2 cup water
1/2 cup raisins
1/2 cup natural sweetener
1/2 cup chopped pecans or walnuts (optional)
2 tsp baking powder
1/2 tsp baking soda
1/2 tsp cinnamon
1/4 tsp nutmeg

Preheat oven to 350. Mix flour, sugar, baking powder, baking soda, cinnamon, and nutmeg together in a large bowl.
Add pumpkin, water, raisins, and nuts. Mix completely. Drop tablespoons onto a baking sheet. Bake 15 minutes, until bottoms are lightly browned. Remove from oven and let stand 2 minutes. Carefully remove from baking sheet with a spatula and place on a rack to cool.

Rainbow Delight
Serves 6

2 apples, grated
2 carrots, grated
2/3 cup shredded coconut
1/2 cup raisins
1/2 cup chopped walnuts

Toss all ingredients together in a bowl and serve.

Green Juicing and Blending

The primary form of dietary supplementation on this diet is in the form of green juicing because it is a way of getting highly concentrated nutrients from high-nutrient plant foods into your system. Consult the *Green Juicing* section under *Sample Recipes* for a variety of recipes. If you do not have a juicer or cannot afford one, you can take the recipes to a local juice bar and they can make them for you. Be sure to call to make sure they have the right ingredients. It's important that you drink the juice right after it is made because it will lose much of its potency if you have it sit around too long.

I would recommend that you consume juiced drinks on an occasional basis, in addition to your regular meals. It is an optional component of the diet.

Wheatgrass is also an excellent dietary supplement. Again, you can have it juiced for you at most natural foods markets and juice bars. It is very strong-smelling due to the chlorophyll, but goes down easier than it smells. Until you get used to it, take an ounce a day, then increase that to two ounces a day. If you want to grow and juice your own wheatgrass, there are resources on the internet that can help you.[1] Health clinics swear by wheatgrass as a dietary supplement and it has been used for well over 30 years.[2] A number of recent scientific studies are starting to bear out these claims.[3] Women who are pregnant or breast feeding should not use wheatgrass.

Ann Wigmore is the woman who introduced wheatgrass to the world and she reversed her own cancer using a natural foods diet with supplementation – after doctors had declared her terminal.

Although she was big on juicing, later in her life she was turning against it and leaning more toward blending because juicing is not the way food is found in

---

[1] A good place to start: www.sproutman.com.

[2] See The Wheatgrass Book, Ann Wigmore.

[3] Shyam R et al., Wheat grass supplementation decreases oxidative stress in healthy subjects: a comparative study with spirulina [letter to the editor]. J Altern Complement Med. 13(8):789-791; Marsili V, Calzuola I, Gianfranceschi GL, Nutritional relevance of wheat sprouts containing high levels of organic phosphates and antioxidant compounds. J Clin Gastroenterol. 2004 Jul;38(6 Suppl):S123-6; Peryt B et al., Mechanism of antimutagenicity of wheat sprout extracts. Mutat Res. 269(2):201-215; Bar-Sela G, Tsalic M, Fried G, Goldberg H, Wheat grass juice may improve hematological toxicity related to chemotherapy in breast cancer patients: a pilot study. Nutr Cancer. 58(1):43-8; Marawaha RK et al., Wheat grass juice reduces transfusion requirement in patients with thalassemia major: a pilot study. Indian Pediatr.41(7):716-20; Fernandes CJ & O'Donovan DJ, Natural antioxidant therapy for patients with hemolyticanemia. Indian Pediatr. 42: 618-619; Pole SN, Wheat grass juice in thalassemia. Indian Pediatr. 43(1):79-80; Ben-Arye E et al., Wheat grass juice in the treatment of active distal ulcerative colitis: a randomized double-blind placebo-controlled trial. Scand J Gastroenterol. 37(4):444-449.

nature. The primary problem with juicing is that it leaves most of the fiber in the food behind and fiber is critical to not only fighting cancer, but also any other disease.

This is the primary problem with too much juicing – you eliminate the fiber and other cancer-fighting nutrients when you throw out the pulp. This is the reason we refer to juicing as optional supplementation. There are clinics which use nothing but juicing when treating cancer patients, for example, and they have had success. I would argue, however, that their success rates would be higher if they used juicing as a supplement, not the main course.

Unlike juicing, blending includes the whole food, as nothing is left behind. In fact, blending can be part of your every day diet and is an excellent way to get more green vegetables into your meals. Because green blending is very concentrated, you need to add small amounts of semi-sweet vegetables to them, such as carrots, apples or tomatoes, in order to make them more palatable. Consult the *Blending* section under *Sample Recipes* for a variety of delicious recipes. You can also find hundreds by searching the internet.

Green Juicing

Green juicing is an excellent way to get concentrated nutrients into your system. The lack of fiber is the trade-off with juicing and because of that, we recommend you juice only once a day. If you do not have a juicer or cannot afford one, you can skip juicing altogether. Or visit your local natural foods store or juice bar and have them make the recipes below.

You can get a basic juicer for $100 to $150. You can also get much more expensive models, such as a Green Star juicer (www.greenstar.com), which actually presses the produce, instead of grinding it. This creates less heat, which increases the juice's quality.

Insofar as directions are concerned, they are the same for all recipes. Cut the ingredients so they will fit into your juicer, juice all ingredients and mix together! If you find the taste too strong, add another carrot or slice of apple.

Green tops, such as the tops of carrots, should always be included in the juicing.

There are an infinite variety of combinations, so please feel free to experiment with different ingredients, depending on what's in the frig!

Cabbage and Celery
3 medium carrots
1 stalk of celery
1/2 green apple
1/4 head of cabbage

Carrot and Cabbage
3-4 Carrots
1-2 Celery stalks
Small wedge cabbage

Cabbage, Beet and Kiwis
2 large kiwis
1 beet (with greens)
1/2 head cabbage

Cucumber, Carrot and Beet
3 carrots
1/2 cucumber
1/2 beet with the greens

Garden Variety
6-8 tomatoes
3-4 green onions
2 carrots
2 stalks celery
1/2 green pepper
1/2 bunch spinach
1/2 bunch parsley

Green Soup
1 leaf collard green, chopped
2 stalks celery
1 leaf kale
1 large tomato
2 cloves garlic
2 pieces scallions, chopped
1/4 cup lemon juice, freshly squeezed
1/4 tsp cayenne pepper

Roll garlic in kale and collard leaf and push through juicer hopper with tomato and celery. Pour mixture into a blender. Add lemon juice and mix. Add cayenne pepper. Mix and adjust to taste. Serve with chopped scallion sprinkled on top of soup.

Renewal
8 large carrots
5 celery stalks
5 radishes
1 large green apple
1 cup cranberries
1/2 large beet
1/2 turnip
1/2 parsnip
1/4 rutabaga
1/8 head red cabbage

Spinach and Celery Delight
4 large spinach leaves
3 stalks celery
2 large carrots
1/2 cup parsley
1/2 beet root
1/2 cup alfalfa sprouts

Spinach, Celery and Asparagus
3 celery stalks
2 asparagus stalks
1 large tomato
Handful of spinach

Sky High Veggies
6 Brussels sprouts
4 medium sweet potatoes (without skin)
4 medium carrots
1 broccoli stalk
1 garlic clove pressed
1 cucumber

The Ultimate
3 carrots
3 collard leaves
2 celery stalks
2 beets
2 garlic cloves
1 turnip
1/2 bunch spinach
1/2 head cabbage
1/2 onion
1/4 bunch parsley

Tomato Juice #1
 (can also be blended)
6 tomatoes
1 cup beet leaves, chopped
1 slice lemon

Tomato Juice #2
 (can also be blended)
4 ripe tomatoes
1 cup green lettuce, packed

V-11 Juice
3 stalks of celery
2 kale leaves
1 head of romaine lettuce
1 cucumber
1 green apple
1 handful cilantro or parsley
1 handful of fennel (use stalk as well)
1 clove garlic
1-2 carrots
1/4 papaya
Handful of spinach leaves

Green Blending (smoothies)

Green blending (smoothies) is an excellent and easy ways to get more green vegetables into your diet. The basic difference between blending and juicing is that you keep everything in foods when you blend them, particularly the fiber, which is extremely important when fighting cancer.

The recipes below are simply suggestions. Feel free to substitute or add ingredients, depending on what you have handy. You can easily adjust smoothies to suit your taste as well. After they are blended, taste a little and if it isn't right, add more ingredients. Smoothies are an excellent way to start the day.

Most ordinary blenders should do the job, but if they don't you can get a very good high-speed blender for less than $100. Vita-Mix is the top of the line and if you get into smoothies, you may want to invest in one of these, or a comparable blender, such as Blendtec.

The directions are the same for all smoothies: simply throw everything into the blender (some ingredients will have to be peeled, of course) and blend until smooth.

Smoothie #1
10 mint leaves
2 cups spinach
3 bananas
2 tbsp carob powder (optional)
1 tsp ground flaxseed
1 cup water

Smoothie #2
2 stalks of celery
2 bananas
2 pears
1 green apple
1 handful spinach
1 tsp ground flaxseed
1 cup water

Smoothie #3
1 handful collard green leaves
1 kale leaf

1 handful mint
4 bananas
1 tsp ground flaxseed
1/2 cup water

Smoothie #4
5 kale leaves
4 apples
1 tsp ground flaxseed
1/2 lemon juiced
1/2 cup water (or to taste)

Smoothie #5
2 cups arugula
2 mangoes
1 handful of spinach
1 tsp ground flaxseed
1 cup water

Smoothie #6
6 kale leaves
3 large bananas
1 handful chard leaves
1 tsp ground flaxseed
1 cup water

Smoothie #7
1 pink grapefruit
1 cucumber
1 lime
1 slice pineapple
1 tsp ground flaxseed
1/2 bunch cilantro
Pinch of cinnamon

Smoothie #8
5 mustard green leaves
2 celery sticks
1 tsp ground flaxseed
1/2 lime juiced
1/2 red onion
1/4 bunch of fresh basil
2 cups of water

Smoothie #9
5 kale leaves
3 cloves garlic
1 cup tomatoes
1 tsp ground flaxseed
1/2 bunch dill
1/2 lime juice
2 cups of water

Smoothie #10
5 kale leaves
3 apples
1 tsp ground flaxseed
1/2 lemon juiced
2 cups of water

Smoothie #11
3 cups red grapes
2 handfuls baby Spinach
1 handful parsley
1 tsp ground flaxseed
2 cups of water

Smoothie #12
3 large handfuls baby spinach
3 bananas
1 tsp ground flaxseed
2 cups of water

Smoothie #13
4 large bananas
2 large handfuls of kale
1 small handful of parsley
1 handful of baby spinach
1 tsp ground flaxseed
2 cups of water

Smoothie #14
2 handfuls baby spinach
1 celery stalk
1 handful parsley

1 Granny Smith apple
1/4 tsp ginger powder (or better 1/2 inch ginger)
1 tsp ground flaxseed
2 cups water

Smoothie #15
4 large ripe bananas
2 large handfuls of kale
1 small handful of parsley
1 handful of baby spinach
1 tsp ground flaxseed
2 cups of water

Smoothie #16
2 pears
2 celery stalks
1 cucumber
1 lemon
1 cup spinach
1 tsp ground flaxseed
1/2 inch ginger
1 cup water

Smoothie #17
1 bunch bok choy
1 banana
1 pear
2 celery stalks
1 tsp ground flaxseed
1 1/2 cup water

Smoothie #18
2 stalks collard greens
1 piece ginger
1 stalk celery
1/2 pineapple (or 1 pear or 1 apple)
1/2 bunch cilantro

Smoothie #19
2 leaves collard greens
2 stalks celery
1 tomato
2 cloves garlic
1 green apple

Food Lists

The following are lists of foods to provide you with suggestions and to also show you the wide variety of foods that available with the RAVE Diet.

Breads

(whole wheat only)

Bagel
Bread - Italian
Bread - French
Bread - pumpernickel
Bread - whole wheat
Bread - rye - American - light
Bread - mixed whole grain
Bread - pita

Bread - oatmeal and bran
Corn taco shells - organic
Muffin - English
Roll - homemade
Spelt and sprouted grain breads
Sprouted whole wheat

Fruits

Apple
Apricot
Avocado
Bananas
Blackberries
Blueberries
Boysenberries
Breadfruit
Carambola
Carissa
Cherimoya
Cherries
Cranberry sauce
Dates
Elderberries
Figs
Gooseberries
Grapefruit
Grapes
Guavas

Kiwifruit
Lemons
Limes
Loganberries
Longans
Loquats
Lychees
Mangos
Melons - cantaloupe
Melons - casaba
Melons - honeydew
Mulberries
Nectarines
Oranges
Papayas
Passion fruit
Peaches
Pears
Persimmons
Pineapple

Pitanga
Plantains
Plums
Pomegranates
Pricklypears
Prunes
Pummelo
Quinces
Raisins
Raspberries
Roselle
Sapodilla
Sapotes
Soursop
Strawberries
Tamarinds
Tangerines
Watermelon

Nuts and Seeds
For nuts, get the unsalted and roasted or raw (preferably raw)

Almonds

Beech

Brazil

Breadfruit

Cashews

Chestnuts

Coconut

Filbert/hazel

Hickory

Macadamia

Peanut butter – (make your own)

Peanuts

Pecans

Pine nuts

Pistachio

Pumpkin/squash seeds

Sesame seeds

Soybean kernels

Sunflower seeds

Walnut

Walnuts

Pasta
Organic soy pasta

Spaghetti – whole wheat

Spelt pasta

Lentil pasta

Quinoa pasta

Whole wheat pasta

Vegetables
Alfalfa seeds - sprouted

Amaranth

Artichokes

Asparagus

Balsam pear

Bamboo shoots

Beans - Great Northern

Beans - green

Beans - snap - yellow/wax

Beans - black

Beans - French

Beans - adzuki

Beans - garbanzo

Beans - green

Beans - lima

Beans - mung

Beans - navy

Beans - red kidney beans

Beans - small white

Beets

Beet greens

Broccoli

Brussels sprouts

Burdock root

Cabbage - savoy

Cabbage - celery

Cabbage - common

Cabbage - red

Cabbage - white mustard

Carrot

Cauliflower

Celery - pascal

Chard - Swiss

Chicory greens

Chickpeas

Chinese vegetables mixed

Chives

Collards

Corn

Cress

Cucumber

Dandelion greens

Eggplant
Endive
Escarole
Fennel
Garlic
Ginger root
Gourd - white flowered
Hummus
Jerusalem artichokes
Kale
Kohlrabi
Leeks
Lentils
Lettuce - iceberg
Lettuce - red leaf
Lettuce - romaine
Lettuce – butter head
Lotus root
Miso - fermented soybeans
Mung bean sprouts
Mushrooms
Mustard greens
Natto - fermented soybeans
Chestchinese
Okra
Onions - mature
Onions - young green
Parsley
Parsnips
Peas - edible podded

Peas - blackeye/cowpeas
Peas - snow pea pods
Peas – split green
Peppers - sweet
Peppers - hot chili
Poi - taro root product
Potato
Pumpkin
Radishes
Rutabaga
Seaweed - spirulina
Seaweed - kelp (kombu)
Shallots
Soybeans - sprouted
Soybeans - green
Spinach
Squash - acorn
Squash - zucchini
Squash - butternut
Squash - summer
Sweet potato
Taro leaf
Taro root
Tomatoes
Turnip greens
Turnips
Water chestnuts
Watercress
Yam - mountain - Hawaii
Zucchini

Whole Grains

Amaranth	Kamut flakes	Spelt flakes
Pearled barley	Matzos	Steel cut oats
Barley flakes	Matzo meal	Teff
Basmati rice (brown)	Millet	Wehani rice
Buckwheat	Popcorn – air popped	Wheat, cracked
Bulgur	Quinoa	Wheat flakes
Couscous	Rice - brown	Wheat germ
Cornmeal	Rolled oats	Wild rice
Cracked wheat	Rye	
Kamut – whole grain	Spelt	

References

For other books, articles and references beyond those cited in the footnotes, please visit www.RaveDiet.com.

Recipe Index

Index